THE RACE VARIABLE

Race, Inequality, and Health

RIH

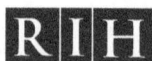

RACE, INEQUALITY, AND HEALTH

Edited by
Samuel Kelton Roberts Jr. and Michael Yudell

The Race, Inequality, and Health series explores how forms of racialization have created a wide range of phenomena, from producing inequities in health and healthcare to inspiring social movements around health. The goal of this series is to publish field-defining works across history, the social sciences, the biological sciences, and public health that deepen our understanding of how claims about race and race difference have affected health and society.

The Race Variable

HOW STATISTICAL PRACTICES REINFORCE INEQUALITY

Jay S. Kaufman

Columbia University Press
New York

Columbia University Press
Publishers Since 1893
New York Chichester, West Sussex
cup.columbia.edu

Copyright © 2026 Columbia University Press
All rights reserved

Cataloging-in-Publication Data is available from the Library of Congress.

ISBN 9780231213622 (hardback)
ISBN 9780231213639 (trade paperback)
ISBN 9780231559942 (ebook)

LCCN 2025024301

Cover design: Elliott S. Cairns

GPSR Authorized Representative: Easy Access System Europe,
Mustamäe tee 50, 10621 Tallinn, Estonia, gpsr.requests@easproject.com

For my father, who got me to care about numbers,
and my mother, who got me to care about people

Les fortes sottises sont souvent faites, comme les grosses cordes, d'une multi-
tude de brins. Prenez le câble fil à fil, prenez séparément tous les petits motifs
déterminants, vous les cassez l'un après l'autre, et vous dites: *Ce n'est que cela!*
Tressez-les et tordez-les ensemble, c'est une énormité.

—VICTOR HUGO, *LES MISÉRABLES* (1862)

Contents

Acknowledgments

This book arises from many years of teaching and research devoted to the epidemiology of racial and ethnic health disparities. My first published scientific paper, written while I was still a doctoral student, sought a new paradigm for conceptualizing and analyzing these inequalities.[1] That was 1995, and in the 30 years that followed, I have tried to keep chipping away at the questions posed in that first paper. While I can't claim to have solved all the problems I identified in that first salvo, I do feel that I have learned a few things along the way. This book is an attempt to share some of those insights.

Sherman James, my doctoral thesis supervisor at the University of Michigan, first focused my attention on race and ethnicity as the most intriguing and beguiling of the social dimensions shaping population health. His work and his mentorship showed me how to approach the topic with rigor and sensitivity, but most importantly, he instilled in me a deep appreciation for the ornate tapestry of human culture and identity and how much meaning these provide us. Concurrently, Jim Koopman in the same department passed along an enduring respect for epidemiological and statistical methodology and my first taste of formal causal inference. These parallel concerns for social justice and quantitative reasoning were further nurtured during a postdoctoral position with Richard Cooper at Loyola Stritch School of Medicine, where more advanced statistical training was provided by Dan McGee. Richard became my most regular collaborator over the decades that followed and a constant source of wisdom and guidance in my life. His untimely passing in April 2024 means that he won't see a book that he did so much to directly influence through his many years of unwavering support.

My first substantive publications on methods for racial and ethnic health disparities were collaborations with my Loyola colleagues, along with some additional direction and advice from Ken Rothman and Hal Morgenstern. After Loyola, I spent a few fallow years as a hospital epidemiologist in Charlotte, North Carolina, before landing an academic position at University of North Carolina at Chapel Hill. There I had the good fortune to be expertly mentored by David Savitz, along with daily methods drills from Charlie Poole. In Chapel Hill, I also learned the most important academic scam, which is that the good students teach you more than you teach them. I was lucky to have advisees who gave me back more than I could ever give them and who became lifelong colleagues, including Lynne Messer, Rich MacLehose, and Anjum Hajat. In 2008, I migrated north to McGill University in Montreal and there continued a run of students who surpassed me, including Tarik Benmarhnia, Corinne Riddell, Hailey Banack, Jeremy Labrecque, and Mabel Carabali, all graduating into treasured friends and collaborators.

Throughout my career, I have benefited greatly from so many generous colleagues in epidemiology and public health who shared their good ideas, gently shot down my bad ones, and served as tireless sounding boards for all my rants and as patient correctives for my misguided efforts. These include my close collaborators at McGill: Sam Harper, Ari Nandi, Nick King, Erin Stumpf, and Seungmi Yang, as well as other mentors, friends, and coauthors who help keep me in line on these issues, including Arnaud Chiolero, Heejung Bang, Maria Glymour, Sander Greenland, Ghassan Hamra, Jim Hanley, Miguel Hernán, Ashley Hirai, Jon Huang, Kerry Keyes, Mike Kramer, Barbara Laraia, Bev Rockhill Levine, Andy Long, Joanna Merckx, Bill Miller, Carles Muntaner, Thu Nguyen, Michael Oakes, Pat O'Campo, Robert Platt, David Richardson, Les Roberts, Enrique Schisterman, Andreas Stang, Steve Stovitz, Daniel Westreich, and Allen Wilcox.

Another crucial platform for collective dialogue on racial and ethnic disparities has been the RACEGEN listserv set up twenty years ago by Jonathan Kahn, Troy Duster, and Duana Fullwiley. This forum has provided me a highly supportive collection of people around the world with similar intellectual interests. I am especially grateful to the continuing education in human genetics received there from Richard Cooper, Joe Graves, and Jon Marks and for the sharing of news, critiques from various disciplinary angles, the periodic kvelling over new books and papers, and the general camaraderie of an intentional community of humane and principled scholars. Among these I mourn the recent loss of Lundy Braun, a role model for careful and impactful work at the intersection of race and medicine.

The bulk of the writing for this book was accomplished during a yearlong sabbatical generously provided by McGill University in 2022–2023, during which time I relocated with my family to Perpignan in Catalogne Nord. My thanks to Maria Melchior at Institut Pierre Louis d'Epidémiologie et de Santé Publique, INSERM, for hosting that stay officially, albeit at a distance. Stephen Wesley at Columbia University Press was a friendly but appropriately insistent editor. He must have worn the paint off of several delete keys but always had an encouraging word to offer, even while he was mercilessly culling most of mine.

I am indebted to Katy Li, who provided invaluable assistance to me in the preparation of the figures used throughout the book. I also must thank Steve Stovitz, who generously read through a draft and was not shy about telling me what worked and what didn't. Three other external reviewers arranged through the publisher provided valuable suggestions anonymously.

Needless to say, the liberty to sit and write eighty thousand words is made possible only by ignoring other things that one should be doing instead, and so my biggest thanks have to be reserved for the cheerful forbearance of my wife and children: Isabelle, Amelia, Julian, Louis, and Sol.

THE RACE VARIABLE

Introduction

O pen any American newspaper, any government report, or any quantitative academic article in the social or biomedical sciences, and you will encounter presentations of racial and ethnic disparities. This focus arises naturally out of the history of the United States, whose European settlers violently displaced an indigenous population, then added millions of Africans through centuries of transatlantic slavery, and later grew through vigorous immigration from all over the world. We find similar concerns about demographic inequalities all over the world, in societies formed by extensive immigration like the United Kingdom and Singapore; in countries that inherited substantial populations from the Atlantic slave trade, such as Brazil and Colombia; and in countries with prominent Indigenous populations, such as Canada, Chile, New Zealand, and Australia.

These multiracial, multiethnic societies are legitimately concerned about equity between their constituent subpopulations, especially in economic and social conditions as well as health and longevity. Most of these countries experienced long periods of legal disempowerment of some racialized populations, from the outright genocide of Native Americans to the legal regimes of racial preference under Jim Crow and Apartheid. Governments, academics, and health systems have a sincere and legitimate interest in documenting and ameliorating the inequalities produced by this systematic discrimination. Hence, there is relentless attention on the range and magnitude of such gaps, the trends across time, and the success of social policy interventions to achieve greater equity. The intentions are noble.

But the documentation, measurement, and dissection of these disparities is essentially a *statistical* activity, and that is where the trouble starts. This somewhat more technical aspect of the problem has received less attention, perhaps because most normal people are not especially interested in or fond of statistics as a discipline. The purpose of this book is to engage with this problem head on: How do we measure, assess, quantify, and decompose racial and ethnic disparities in the service of this legitimate public interest? My contention is that most of the time we don't do this very thoughtfully or effectively, and so a great deal of misunderstanding arises from these deficiencies. I believe that we can do better, if we are willing to give some thought to how the data are managed and analyzed, and that the benefit of doing so will be a much clearer depiction of existing injustices.

The quantitative study of racial and ethnic inequality naturally begins with definitions—that is, how a dynamic process of lumping and splitting forms a tractable number of groups that we may monitor for equity. This is a process that is overtly historical and political, while at the same time subject to bureaucratic decisions that can be perplexing and inconsistent. Then, for any domain, there is the measure of an outcome of interest, whether economic, social, or biomedical, and the comparison between groups to assess how they differ from one another. Were it to stop there, the problem would be much simpler, and this book would be much shorter. But a central theme that pervades this book is that we do not generally rely on these direct comparisons between the outcomes of racial and ethnic groups. Instead, we almost always make statistical *adjustments* to massage these disparities, supposedly for better specificity, clarity, or insight. These adjustments make statistics a powerful tool for data analysis and underly much of the success of modern science across all quantitative disciplines. But mindful of the equity concerns that are the underlying motivation for the study of disparities, my contention is that these statistical adjustments of racial and ethnic disparities are not always well-founded, are not always applied thoughtfully or validly, and in practice do much to confuse and obscure the truth and hobble even the most well-intentioned public policies.

Some blame lies in the application of techniques that were designed for other purposes, for example statistical models for the testing of drugs versus placebos in clinical trials. The statistical foundations for valid adjustments of racial and ethnic disparities are not widely discussed or taught, and this hobbles efforts to achieve a consensus about the best practices for quantitative social science. Some blame lies in misunderstandings by researchers, who come to apply some adjustments in routine ways while they lose track of the underlying motivations for these maneuvers. Some blame lies with the news media, who often process academic work for popular consumption by ignoring important caveats and assumptions and, frankly, even sometimes misinterpret results. Some blame lies with the politicized nature of the discourse on social inequalities, which exploits ambiguities in the presentation of statistical evidence to support ideologically driven narratives.

This topic is inherently a technical one, and a critique of statistical tools necessarily requires some willingness to engage with the mathematical foundations of these procedures. I have written the book assuming no formal background in statistics on behalf of the reader, and it is my hope that any interested reader can appreciate the arguments with minimum anguish. Mathematical notation is kept to a minimum, and when necessary, I make every attempt to explain the symbols and their interpretation. There is a fair amount of algebra but only with elementary operations at a grade-school level. The notion of a statistical model is fundamental to this discussion, and the most important of these is the linear regression model, which is the workhorse of almost all adjustment techniques discussed in the book (figure 0.1). This is just a mathematical procedure for fitting a straight line through a cloud of data points to determine a measure of central tendency, an average behavior of one variable in relation to another. The fitting of this

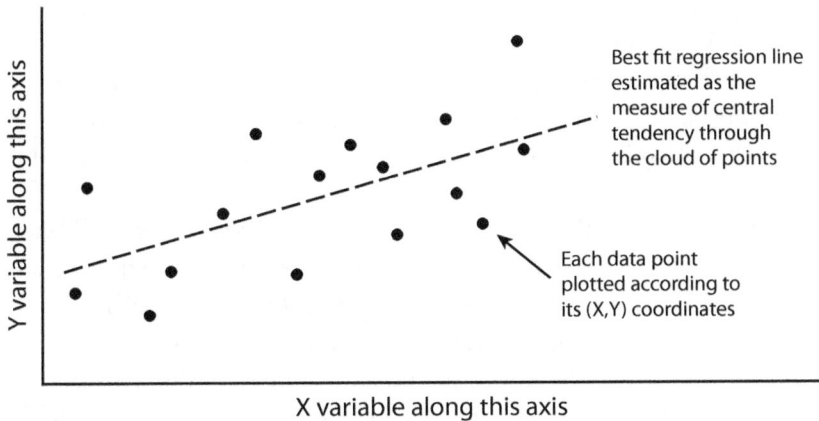

Figure 0.1 Linear regression model for the relationship between two variables: X and Y.

model is generally accomplished with software that allows the parameters to be generated automatically with the press of a button. This ease of use has greatly expanded the application of these models but, at the same time, made analysts a bit lazy about thinking through what the model is doing, how the estimates can be validly interpreted, and what the exact problem is that's supposedly being solved.

To demonstrate what this looks like in practice, consider a routine example of a reported racial contrast. The American College of Surgeons recommends drug screening of trauma patients but sets no specific guidelines for doing so. A recently published study using a sample of over 85,000 injured American adolescents reported that although 21.8 percent of all patients were screened for drugs, adjusted odds of screening were 13 percent higher for Black compared to white adolescents and 75 percent higher for American Indian adolescents.[1] But maybe there were other characteristics of these individuals that explained their disparate treatment, like the type of injury or their insurance status. To address that possibility, the authors *adjusted* for a long list of factors using a regression model like that described earlier. How do the investigators select these factors and carry out this adjustment? What are the assumptions and limitations of this maneuver? What can go wrong (and usually does) in the modeling and the interpretation? These are some of the questions that I will attempt to address in the pages that follow. The problem of careless statistical practice in social and biomedical sciences is not unique to the realm of racial and ethnic disparities, but in this domain, there are strong prior expectations and compelling mythologies that can often drive the narrative far beyond what is warranted by the data. Sensationalist journalism doesn't help—in fact, it often amplifies results and filters out important caveats. But races and ethnicities are identities, and thus, it is inevitable that researchers, journalists, and readers all feel some sense of connection and familiarity with the categories. We all have some skin in the game when it comes to representing advantaged and disadvantaged statuses against one another.

Another theme of this book, however, is that the expectation of objectivity in this realm is itself somewhat misguided because the optimal adjustment strategies in any given situation will depend on values, judgments, and priorities that are not and cannot be completely objective. Statistics is taught as a branch of mathematics, with proofs and theorems, as though analysis of data relies on pure impassionate logic alone. In its abstract theory, this may be true. But once statistics is applied to social phenomena, that objectivity quickly evaporates. Model selection can no longer proceed algorithmically according to mathematical principles alone. Adjustment acts as a form of imposed morality in which the statistical model turns *what is* into *what should be*. Entering that conjectural space requires ethical considerations on which all are not apt to agree.

There are many cited examples in this book, like the earlier example of drug screening, largely drawn from the recent published literature across social and biomedical sciences. Mostly I offer these examples so that I can critique their analysis or interpretation. But I must stress that these articles are not selected for any unique transgressions but rather because they are broadly representative of common limitations and errors that are everywhere in the work published by public agencies, academics, and research organizations. They are merely convenient examples of widespread habits. In this sense, I hope that the authors of these examples will not feel personally attacked. The examples are selected for being completely normative in their strengths and deficiencies, which is why they are such useful illustrations. Most examples are also from the United States, merely because of its dominance in social science and biomedical research as well as its persistent commitment to racial and ethnic classification in all public records, facilitating the documentation of disparities in every facet of life and death.

Neither should these critiques make us abandon the measurement and investigation of racial inequities. I do wish that we lived in a world in which these classification, documentation, and analysis activities were unnecessary, but sadly we do not. Our world is still too full of racial and ethnic injustice, and not monitoring this, not studying it, and not understanding it will not make it go away. Our hope lies in doing things better, not doing nothing at all.

CHAPTER I

<hr>

What Is This Thing Called Race?

This is a book about racial and ethnic disparities and the misuse of race in statistics. So we must necessarily begin with an examination of the construct of race itself. What is race? What are the historical roots of this idea? And how has it arrived in the datasets we use today? The question of what the identities of race and ethnicity mean historically, anthropologically, politically, and biologically is a longstanding problem that occupies many books,[1] and indeed even entire encyclopedias.[2] We can only scratch the surface here, but it is a necessary first step before we can consider how disparities are managed statistically.

Over the course of human history, there have been innumerable variations of the within-versus-between distinction among groups of people and endless ingenuity in the use of physical and cultural traits to cement such divisions.[3] Old World societies imbued all national and ethnic distinctions with at least a tinge of essentialism, as with the stereotypical traits of the French, Italians, Germans, and so on. What emerged in the post-Columbian world of colonial conquest and industrial-scale slave trading, however, was a categorical *continental* distinction, a world made up of Europeans, Africans, Asians, Americans. These are the "varieties" of *Homo sapiens* proposed by Linnaeus.[4] This broad grouping implied natural branches of humanity, like subspecies, and it served to justify, among other things, a brutal and perpetual chattel slavery for Africans in the New World. Categorical race as natural law became a practical social necessity in a land of mixed European heritage, especially one that was economically dependent on kidnapped people from across the ethnically diverse Atlantic coast of Africa.[5] Extreme even among systems of slavery, the American version transcended typical "us versus them" distinctions because it required first Native Americans and then Africans to be scientifically certified as subhuman.[6]

By the latter half of the twentieth century, the United States had become the world's dominant engine of social and biomedical research, which served to export its extreme culture of racialized social arrangements as a global social and scientific norm. An idiosyncratic American view of race that had evolved to suit the needs of slave owners, and later massaged through Reconstruction and Jim Crow, was broadcast around the world in film, popular culture, and scientific practice. Consider the "one-drop rule," by which mixed-race individuals were assigned unambiguously to the inferior caste. This had not always been the norm in the United States and even less so elsewhere. In the Spanish colonial tradition, for example, mixed-race individuals took on a distinctly intermediate social categorization, perpetuated in the *mestizo* or *pardo* classifications found in Mexico and Brazil even today.[7] Many American states also enacted fractional categories like *mulatto*, *quadroon*, and *octoroon* in the late nineteenth century, although without formal criteria so that the genealogical precision implied by such terms was illusory. The United States eventually evolved toward a more rigidly binary system, legally enshrining the doctrine of *hypodescent* in the early twentieth century.[8] Because the United States exerted such an overwhelming cultural influence after World War II, this notion, as opposed to the graded racial hierarchies of Latin America, became more universally normative. A consequence of this hegemony of U.S. race culture is that few people anywhere in the world would question, say, the status of Barack Obama, the child of a white mother, as a "Black" American president.[9]

And yet classification was never a simple matter. Racial boundaries are sociopolitical conventions without any objective justifications, so they were always stretched and contested by the conflicting interests and priorities of the day. Consider the Virginia aristocracy, who claimed to be descended from the early Jamestown settler John Rolfe and his wife Pocahontas. In Virginia, the one drop rule enshrined in law until 1967 would have banned these descendants from marrying a white person in the state. But that just wouldn't do. Hence, lawmakers added the "Pocahontas Exception" to the antimiscegenation laws in the state.[10] States passed laws that constantly contradicted one another on the minimum criteria for achieving whiteness and were, in any case, fundamentally unenforceable without sophisticated genea-logical records. Census takers classified people by visual inspection without any formal procedures, and people sometimes won new racial classifica-tions in court based on their social presentations alone. This was the case for Ralph Dupas, who petitioned for a new birth certificate in Louisiana to demonstrate that he was white so that he could compete in segregated sporting events. The state supreme court ruled in 1960 that even though he clearly had Black parents, "the principle of law with respect to degree of proof required in the present case depends largely on whether [Dupas] has been accepted as a member of the white or Caucasian race during his lifetime . . . [and] evidence on this point seems overwhelming."[11]

Although state legislatures and judges sometimes reached contradictory decisions on how to sort people, the federal government maintained no overt standards throughout most of its history. Since the first official census in 1790, racial and ethnic categories changed regularly, often in response to direct political mobilization or in reaction to social pressures such as mass immigration.[12] It was only in 1977 that official categories for statistical pur-poses were formally systematized by the federal government with the adop-tion of the U.S. Office of Management and Budget (OMB) Directive 15.[13] The directive established definitions for racial and ethnic groups to be used in federal administration, but the document itself warned that its classifica-tions "should not be interpreted as being scientific or anthropological in nature." Like the famously telescoping *New Yorker* cartoon of the world seen from Manhattan, OMB Directive 15 also broadcast America's geographical chauvinism. For example, it defined the "Asian or Pacific Islander" race to include everything between Pakistan and the coast of California, capturing unrelated peoples across roughly half of the earth's surface and compris-ing roughly half of all human beings. Or consider the directive's definition of the "Black race" as people descended from "the black racial groups of Africa," suggesting that "Black" and "race" are such primordial constructs that their definitions can only be circular. Directive 15 identified only a single ethnicity for government purposes, "Hispanic," which it defined as people of Spanish culture or origin, regardless of race.[14]

Twenty years later, in 1997, the Directive 15 guidelines were slightly updated.[15] The revision focused on just two small modifications: splitting the Asian and Pacific Islander category into two, "Asian" and "Native Hawaiian or Other Pacific Islander," and modifying the "Hispanic" ethnicity to "His-panic or Latino." Today, as I write this book in 2024, the guidelines have just changed again, with the major innovation being the splitting off of whites from a new North African and Middle Eastern racial category.[16] Other changes include gathering race and ethnicity in a single question, which means that those identifying as Hispanic or Latino no longer select an additional race category as they could before. The "American Indian or Alaska Native" category has expanded to include all individuals who identify with any of the pre-Columbian peoples of the Americas, finally correcting an oversight of the previous guidelines that offered no place for Indigenous populations from outside the United States like Maya and Aztecs. This new revision is the culmination of an intensely political process, starting with the establishment of the Federal Interagency Technical Working Group on Race and Ethnicity Standards in 2022 and proceeding with public hearings and input from a wide assortment of agencies including the Census Bureau, the National Center for Health Statistics, and the Department of Homeland Security. The OMB announced guiding principles for this process, starting with the premise that "race and ethnicity are sociopolitical constructs and are not an attempt to define race and ethnicity biologically or genetically."[17]

Race, then, is plastic. Throughout history, it has been molded and reconfigured as needed, often for nakedly political reasons. How should we then think about race in the context of statistics, especially in the data through which disparities are estimated, reported, and studied? This book takes as a premise that race and ethnicity are best seen as distinctions of identity, affiliation, and social recognition. The lines between groups might be arbitrary, inconsistent, and malleable. The person who is Black in the United States might not be Black (*preto*) in Brazil but rather mixed (*pardo*). Indeed, one recent survey of Brazilians captured 136 distinct skin color self-descriptions, from *acastanhada* ("somewhat chestnut-colored") to *turva* ("murky").[18] Despite this inevitable chaos of arbitrary lumping and splitting, people do generally have a locally salient identity. And that identity is highly consequential as a determinant of social position, as well as occupation, diet, residential patterns, family formation, and how others treat them. How others treat them is especially important for our purposes when those others are educators, employers, or law enforcement, for instance.[19]

These factors are gateways that control the smoothest paths available in a person's health and social life. They have ramifications for medicine, criminal justice, economics, and sociology. Race does matter, and therefore, it must be recorded and studied by government administrators and social scientists. At the same time, we must always bear in mind that race is a cultural invention, like money or religion. It is an abstract construction with somewhat arbitrary parameters, but it nonetheless dominates our lives because we have invested so much sincere belief in it. In light of this indisputable centrality for social recognition and status, American researchers and government agencies have a compelling interest in monitoring and documenting racial and ethnic disparities in health, education, economic progress, and criminal justice.[20] This is why the OMB must convene the complex process described earlier, in which a huge bureaucracy is guided through the baroque ordinances governing the collection and processing of these data. At the same time, we must acknowledge that by documenting and studying race, we unintentionally reinforce it, perpetuating its hold on us.[21] In contrast, after World War II, the French, having observed with horror how racial classification abetted mass murder, made it illegal for the government to collect such data.[22] The result today is a society just as noxiously racist but without the data to quantify this social harm.[23]

Although race is a cultural invention, biological variation is not. Humans clearly look somewhat different from place to place, even if these traits fall along gradients (referred to by physical anthropologists as *clines*) with no objective cut points.[24] Even when we use a physical trait like skin color as the basis for racial distinctions, it does not necessarily capture biological relatedness. Light skin color is an adaptation to higher latitudes, presumably a consequence of reduced ultraviolet radiation in these environments. Unrelated people who are adapted to similar latitudes therefore have similar skin tones, without necessarily having much else in common, including, for example, dark-skinned people in Melanesia (from which its name evolved) as well as South Asia and the Andes.[25] The race construct that we recognize socially does not correspond to significant biological clustering. Because genes are transmitted through a process involving two humans arranging themselves in close proximity, people tended over most of our history to be genetically similar to those living close by and more distinct from those living far away. This is why local ethnic groups can be genetically clustered in ways that continental races cannot be. Broad racial groupings cannot be especially informative, therefore, and the physical or biological generalizations drawn from them are not all that useful for accurate predictions in fields like psychology, medicine, or sport.

Modern humans spent a quarter of a million years in East and southern Africa, whereas the ancestors of all non-Africans ventured away from that cradle of our species only in the last sixty thousand years or so.[26] This means that almost all of our ancestry is shared broadly across all of humanity and explains why between-group biological differences remain small compared to within-group differences. Although there exists some detectable degree of human genetic variability across continental clusters, this is swamped by the variation *within* each cluster. A genetic variant might therefore be somewhat more or less common in one continental group compared to another, but most variants exist to a greater or lesser extent in all large groups of humans. Some of the continental variation that does exist arose when populations left Africa and did not bring all of the existing human biological variation with them.[27] In addition, humans continually adapt physically to new environments. Because environments are also widely shared across continents, these adaptations occurred in parallel among many unrelated peoples. For example, high-altitude populations are adapted for low-oxygen environments, and this is true equally of Tibetans, Ethiopians, and Bolivians, despite having no notable genetic similarity.[28] Even paradigmatically race-associated traits like sickle cell anemia vary widely within continental groups, occurring at higher prevalence in some populations that we call "white" than in some we call "Black."[29] The ethnicity construct can come closer to the kind of localized ancestry that better captures this history of adaption and isolation, especially for smaller groups, but this is not reflected in the five hundred million people subsumed under the administratively constructed "Hispanic" ethnicity, the only one that is officially recognized by U.S. government agencies.[30]

Given that racial divisions are historical, political, and sociological artifacts, there is obviously no objective way to determine someone's "true" race. As a facet of identity, which is necessarily held internally by a person in a subjective way, the only practical means to ascertain someone's race is to ask them. When a forensic investigator uses physical measurements to "determine" the race of a cadaver, they are only making a best guess about how the person might have identified while alive.[31] Because it is now well known that assignment of race by others is imperfectly correlated with self-identification, it has indeed become common practice to ask people to describe themselves, allowing for the reality that individual responses can and do change over time.[32] A recent study in one large American hospital system showed that almost 7 percent of its pediatric patients changed race at least once over a ten-year period,[33] and about one in eight American children changed their individual race response between the 2000 census and 2010 census.[34] Many people find the categories offered on surveys and official documents to be limiting or irrelevant, and so they simply decline to respond. This is especially true of people with complex identities, such as those of mixed race or those with ethnically discordant parents.[35] This raises the technical dilemma in data analysis of how to manage these instances in which racial or ethnic data are missing because the participant refused to respond to the question.

Both observed and self-reported categorizations of race and ethnicity can be uncomfortable, inconsistent, and incomplete. Because of this dilemma, many medical scientists now propose replacing such reporting with genetic ancestry estimated from DNA.[36] This has become a common procedure, in which a tissue sample is collected and analyzed against a database of samples from populations around the world. At each of many selected locations on the genome, the variant of the donor is compared to the frequency of that variant in the reference populations. For example, if I go to Japan and collect DNA from people there who I believe to represent the native population in some sense,[37] then I have a working reference for the distribution of genetic traits in that population. I have to collect this reference data for all human populations that I might care about, and then I must fit a statistical model that estimates a continuous degree of membership of the sample donor with each of these modeled ancestry populations in my database. Statistical models can also estimate clusters of more closely related populations, based on comparing multidimensional distances across all the different markers used. These modeled clusters then serve as the statistical realization of a race construct.

The popularity of ancestry estimation from DNA for recreational purposes has made this technology widely familiar, and about one in five Americans have already mailed off vials of their spit to discover their heritage through such techniques.[38] But despite the apparent advantages, the connection between this modeled ancestry and the race quantity of fundamental interest is actually quite limited. One clear advantage of using ancestry estimated from genotyping is that people with multiracial identities are no longer forced into endorsing a single racial classification because the DNA test estimates continuous degrees of relatedness to every defined ancestry cluster. The test can also be applied when the individual cannot respond themselves, for example by taking tissue from infants or cadavers. Nonetheless, the results remain a somewhat arbitrary function of the samples collected in the referent database.[39] Which ancestral peoples are sampled? How are representative samples of these people obtained, and how do we know that the people found in the sampled region are the same ones who lived there at the time when the donor was historically connected to that population? After all, the world has never been static; populations have always moved around and mixed over time.

There is also a necessary discrepancy in time for ancestry tests. If a donor's ancestor left Africa five hundred years ago, we would need to compare their sample to a database of DNA from different regions of Africa five hundred years ago and not modern African DNA. The use of contemporary populations as proxies for ancestral populations is a sleight of hand. It seems impossible to know how different those proxies might be, especially because "ancestry" has no explicit time scale in these analyses.[40] Humans spent the vast majority of our history as a species in Africa, so if the tests were not somehow bounded in time, everyone's results would come back overwhelmingly African.

Statistical models such as those used in DNA ancestry testing would ideally be calibrated using samples with known values, but ancestry is an inherently latent quantity that has no specific quantifiable true value. Groupings are arbitrarily defined and the time scale is ignored. The whole idea of precise ancestry *proportions* is patently absurd because we have no known denominator number of ancestors. The results are typically delivered to paying customers with a numerical precision that implies some kind of scientific certitude, but this feigned precision is nothing but a marketing ploy. There is no objective verification of such numbers or their potential errors, nor indeed can we even define a gold standard for what the number should really be in principle.[41]

These commercial ancestry kits and the multidimensional ancestry information they purport to discover might be entertaining, but it is not the race variable we're interested in here. The race variable that is the subject of this book is the one that is used in descriptive analyses of social disparities, especially in fields like medicine, economics, education, and criminal justice. These differences are primarily about social treatment, and this depends much more on a person's perceived race than it does on fractions of biological ancestry. Certainly one's historical lineage is not wholly irrelevant because phenotype places some boundaries on what race people can assert themselves to be. But in famous liminal cases, we generally find that identity trumps biology, and race is much more about culture than it is about DNA. Consider the case of Wayne Joseph, a Black man originally from the segregated parishes of Louisiana who took a DNA test and found he had 0 percent African ancestry.[42] I discuss this issue in somewhat more detail in chapter 6 in the context of measurement error, considering the race variable we find in our datasets and imagining what might be the real underlying information we are trying to capture with that quantity.

Even if we are obligated to collect some racial information to monitor differential social treatment, we can't become complacent about the way that this is done in practice. We must continually reevaluate arguments for the potential benefits versus harms of collecting or not collecting racial identity in specific data sources. And we must keep our minds open to changing how these data are assessed and recorded. For example, how can we better accommodate the growing acceptance of multiple racial identities, the relation of identity to the exploding availability of DNA-based ancestry testing, and the awareness that one's self-identity can differ from the racial characteristics that others perceive? As immigration increases worldwide and almost all countries become more ethnically complex, the significance of these historical notions of race is constantly challenged, and these notions must continually adapt, as they have in the past. Race is a double-edged sword for data science. We can't live with it, and we seemingly can't live without it. It is a long-standing social invention and remains a highly conse-quential one. It demands our attention as a significant force shaping human interactions and institutions. Especially in societies like the United States, with its long history of de jure discrimination and de facto prejudice, ignor-ing the social and historical fact of race is unrealistic and irresponsible. Some even argue that to ignore such a highly informative social marker would be unethical.[43] And yet at the same time, these groupings are scientifically untenable, and paying attention to them risks reinforcing and legitimizing them and their atavistic notions of essentialism and hierarchy. Medicine in particular has a responsibility to eschew folkloric distinctions in favor of scientific ones, through rigorous processes of quantification, experimenta-tion, and evaluation. Race does not meet these standards, and so it ought to fade from use as we increasingly favor personalized, evidence-based tests, algorithms, and procedures that privilege a patient's individual humanity over obsolete and misleading stereotypes.[44]

We might look to ethnicity, rather than race, as a potentially more spe-cific indicator of common cultural experience, language, and geographic origin. But often even these categories are ineffectual. Consider the broad Hispanic ethnicity as implemented in official statistics in the United States. It's a vague hodgepodge of groups that have only the loosest linguistic and cultural commonality. Often categories of ethnicity are so broad that they are hardly more distinct or helpful than race. Both variables are forms of identity, and therefore, they are matters of internal awareness that cannot be objectively verified. But they do operate within some bounds. What I mean is that to adopt an identity that is discordant with the perceptions of others can be a source of considerable social tension.[45] Despite the advent of recreational genetics and its promise to reveal hidden identities, there is no necessary relationship between test results and self-concept. Of course self-concept is malleable, and genetic results can influence them if people believe the results. In practice, however, it seems that commercial ancestry tests tend to reinforce the identities that people already embrace, or else they are dismissed.[46]

This book considers statistical comparisons of racial and ethnic groups. These constructs are overwhelming; they have penetrated all social and scientific domains, from demography to medicine. The lack of an objective or stable demarcation of these groupings does not lessen their real impact on real people. Although the categories and their boundaries may change over time, the existence of disparities does not. There are many concerns about racial and ethnic stratifications and adjustments, and there is always the danger that studying them may legitimize them. They may lead to feelings of fatalism and stigmatization that are real concerns.[47] Although we must be mindful of the ethics of our studies, we cannot ignore such crucial social determinants of health and economic and social well-being. We must proceed thoughtfully and cautiously—but we must proceed.

CHAPTER II

Causality and the Fundamental Challenge
of Observed Correlation

T his chapter considers the potential goals of a statistical analysis:
description, prediction, or causal inference. It is perhaps surprising that scientific authors do not always state clearly their precise
motivations when they construct statistical models to make adjustments and
corrections.[1] This ambiguity of purpose, albeit common, can be catastrophic
for validity because different purposes require distinct statistical considerations and methods.[2] Some scientific projects, including many described
in this book, are *causal* studies. They aim to quantify the magnitude of the
effect of some policy, treatment, or exposure on a chosen outcome quantity.
This chapter reviews some basic ideas about causal inference and how they
might apply to work on racial and ethnic disparities. The statistical methods
for inferring causal relationships were designed with assignable treatments
in mind, such as you would find in an experimental study in a laboratory. If I conduct a study in which participants are assigned to take a pill
that contains either a vitamin or a placebo, every participant is capable of
ingesting either of these treatments. An immediate problem arises if we try
to apply these same methods to relatively fixed demographic characteristics
like race and ethnicity.[3] These cannot usually be assigned in an experiment
because they are identities held deeply by human beings. Nobody can flip
a coin and assign patients in a clinical trial to be Mexican or Asian. This
mismatch—statistical techniques developed for one setting but applied in
another—can be challenging for the assumptions and interpretations of

these procedures. This has led to decades of debate. Before we get into all that, however, let's first review and explain the basic statistical goals and ideas to see how these original intentions affect decisions about modeling and adjustment. Then we can consider how they might apply to the study of racial and ethnic differences.

The first kind of study, and the simplest conceptually, is the purely descriptive study. In this design, the purpose is merely to depict the true state of the world, just as a photograph captures a landscape. In the context of epidemiology, this might be referred to as *surveillance*. For example, if I want to report the number of deaths from COVID-19 in Ohio in 2021, I can examine all death certificates filed for residents of that state in that year and search for mentions of COVID-19 among the causes of death listed on the death certificates. If I can assume that all true deaths are detected and that there are no errors in the assignment of the cause of death, then I simply report this count, without any adjustments or manipulations. Statistical corrections are only needed if I am aware of some coding errors or inaccuracies in reporting. This kind of surveillance is a key public health function because "epidemics" are defined by excess incidence of disease. We can only detect such excesses by establishing a baseline and then monitoring events over time.[4] Descriptive work like this is also common in economics and demography, where governments, banks, or corporations need to know the current state of the world in rich detail based on surveys, censuses, or administrative records.

A descriptive study might involve casting our gaze over the entire population. For example, the United States and many other countries compile a National Death Index, which collects every death certificate that is issued. It is easy to surveil this dataset to describe all deaths in the county in any selected interval of time. But descriptive data can also be based on a random sample rather than measuring every single individual in the population. For example, suppose I needed to know the proportion of Ohio residents who have detectable antibodies to COVID-19 in their blood, indicating that they have experienced a SARS-CoV-2 infection in the past. It is not practical to draw blood from everyone in Ohio, and so this estimated prevalence would have to be extrapolated from a random sample of residents. Still, no adjustments or controls are needed in principle, because the numbers that I am interested in are those that are directly observable; they pertain to the real world at the present time.

Adjustments might only become necessary if something goes wrong, for instance if some people refuse to participate in the survey after they were randomly selected. If such refusals were to occur, my estimate could be *biased*, meaning that the procedure I use is not expected to yield the true value in the whole population. This could happen, for example, if the people who refuse have a higher proportion of past illness, and therefore, my achieved sample would be more healthy than in the general population that I hope to describe. This is referred to as *selection bias* and will be discussed in greater detail in chapter 5. Biases like these are exactly the kinds of situations in which statistical adjustments must be applied. In the case of selection bias, I would hope to use some external information to nudge the estimate back, closer to its true value.[5]

Some surveillance based on random samples also engages in intentional oversampling, usually because there are small groups that warrant special attention. For example, surveys conducted by the Canadian government often oversample the Inuit population. This is because they number only about seventy thousand out of more than forty million Canadians. A simple random sample would include too few to make any definitive statements. So for some small populations of particular interest, like the Inuit, a decision is made in the design of the survey that these groups should be oversampled, which means that the number invited to participate is larger than their representation in the population. Then after the data are collected, the statistical analysis is weighted so that the oversampled observations count proportionately less in any summary of the whole population.[6]

The second kind of study is a prediction about a future outcome. We sometimes refer to these as *prognostic* studies. A doctor who diagnoses a patient with cancer might typically be asked for the probability that this patient will still be alive in five years. This is a question about the real world, yes, but about the real world in the future. So, in contrast to the descriptive study, the outcome cannot be immediately observed. To answer this kind of question requires some kind of statistical model in which data on previous patients—when they were diagnosed and when they died—are used to divine the future of someone in the present. A statistical model is just as the name implies: it is a toy that looks superficially like reality but would never be mistaken for reality, just as you would never fly to Europe in a model airplane. This statistical model makes some simple assumptions about how the different characteristics of previous patients, like age and sex, interact with each other to predict what will happen to the current patient. Once the prediction is made, we can follow up later to see how close the model came to the truth and tweak it as necessary to improve its predictive accuracy in the future. In principle, the more things we measure about the patient, the better is the prediction. We also must assume that the future will operate just like the past. If a new cancer treatment is discovered, for instance, then predictions based on past patients can become outdated. Certain fields like meteorology, medicine, and economics are especially dependent on accurate predictions, but they arise as a crucial analysis in almost all scientific fields. In criminology, for example, there is a great deal of attention devoted to the prediction of recidivism.[7]

The third and final type of study is about causal inference. Suppose one wants to know the effect of a policy or treatment based on a statistical comparison of people, some of whom were treated and some of whom were not treated. This is actually the most common kind of statistical analysis that is reported in the news media, scientific journals, and evidence presented for policymakers. To make some decision about an action like getting a COVID-19 vaccine, I must accurately predict two outcomes: what will happen if I take the vaccine and what will happen if I don't take the vaccine. Then I must consider whether the contrast of those two predicted numbers is compelling for me. Data are necessary for these predictions, and when these data arise from comparisons of people who actively chose to take or not to take the vaccine, one should naturally be concerned that the characteristics of these groups could be different. Variables included in an analysis that are not the treatment or outcome variables are referred to as *covariates*. For example, one important covariate in this example could be age. If older people had more concern about COVID-19 because they know that age is a risk factor for severe disease, then the vaccinated group might be older than the unvaccinated group on average, leading to more deaths in that group. This mixing of effects—because the vaccinated group differs not only in vaccination but also in age—is referred to as *confounding*.

We don't anticipate this problem of confounding in randomized laboratory experiments or controlled clinical trials. In those settings, people are not selecting their own treatments, and so all other characteristics of the participants tend to be balanced across the treatment groups. But in observational studies, which constitute most of the literature in biomedical and social science fields, confounding is always a concern.[8] There is no reason why a confounding bias need only be due to a single covariate—there could be hundreds or thousands of traits that differ between the treated and untreated groups. Moreover, these traits can often be unmeasured or even unmeasurable. Can we ever begin to imagine all of the personality factors that might be involved in the decision to take a vaccine or not? This skepticism about potential confounding is the basis for the oft-repeated warning that "correlation is not causation." That is to say, when treatment or exposure is not under the control of the investigator, then any amount of confounding (i.e., imbalance of other variables) can occur. So, if the observed difference in a study was that vaccinated people had half the death rate, this association alone does not imply that assigning the vaccine to other people would cut their risk of death in half.

Statistical adjustments for confounding often involve splitting up a covariate into its component levels (also called *strata*, from the Latin word for "layers"), then estimating the effect of the treatment within the levels of the covariate, and finally putting those separate estimates back together again. Here's a simple numerical example to demonstrate how this would work. Suppose I conduct that survey on reported COVID-19 vaccination in relation to severe illness. I have eighty people in the study, and the data are provided in table 2.1.

The risk of severe illness in the vaccinated group is 20/40 = 50 percent. The risk of severe illness in the unvaccinated group is also 20/40 = 50 percent. From these two proportions, we can calculate that the observed risk difference is 50 percent − 50 percent = 0. Therefore, based on these observed data, we have no reason to believe that vaccination would be beneficial in relation to this outcome. The difference contrast of 0 between the two risks is the "null" result—the one that corresponds to the absence of any causal effect. If I prefer the ratio-scale contrast, 50 percent/50 percent = 1. Once again, there is no evidence for an effect because the null value for a ratio contrast is 1. We'll discuss these different contrast scales more in chapter 9.

Are we done? That depends. There are other variables that might predict severe disease, such as age. If the assignment of the vaccine was randomized,

TABLE 2.1
Occurrence of severe illness in relation to COVID-19 vaccination status

	Vaccination	No vaccination	Total
Sick	20	20	40
Not sick	20	20	40
Total	40	40	80

we can be confident that the age distributions of the two treatment groups become increasingly similar as the sample size gets larger. This achieved balance of all the other variables is also a function of the sample size. This is because of a probabilistic phenomenon known as the strong law of large numbers. This law guarantees that as a random process is applied to a larger and larger number of observations, it must approach its expected value. For example, a fair coin toss has a probability of landing on heads half the time. But on a single flip, it is impossible to observe 50 percent heads; it must be either heads or tails. And you might not get heads 50 percent of the time in two flips either. Think of a gambling game in which two players are each given a fair coin to toss. They each flip their own coin a set number times, and we will calculate the percentage of heads for each person, and they win a prize if the difference in the two proportions is greater than 0.10. For example, suppose we ask them to each flip their coins ten times. The first player gets six heads out of ten (6/10 = 0.60). The second player gets four heads out of ten (4/10 = 0.40). Because 0.60 − 0.40 = 0.20, and this is greater than 0.10, they win the prize. Table 2.2 shows those probabilities for various numbers of flips between 10 and 100.

As the number of flips increases, the imbalance between the two players must decrease, as each run of flips converges to its expected value of 50 percent, with less and less random deviation. At ten flips, an imbalance as big

TABLE 2.2

Probability of winning a coin flipping game in relation to the number of coin flips by two players

Number of flips	Expected difference in proportion of heads between the two players	Chance of winning the prize
10	0.176	82.4%
20	0.125	63.6%
30	0.103	51.9%
40	0.089	43.4%
60	0.073	31.5%
80	0.063	23.6%
100	0.056	17.9%

as 0.1 between the two proportions will happen most of the time. But once there are more than thirty flips, that magnitude of imbalance happens only about half the time. At a hundred flips, the expected difference between the proportions is down to 0.056, and only 17.9 percent of the time will the difference be bigger than 0.10. This is how randomized trials balance other factors between the two treatment groups and why large trials are more effective in this balancing than small trials.[9]

Our imaginary data do not come from a randomized trial, however, but from a survey, meaning that we had no control over who received a vaccine. We must therefore be concerned that an important risk factor like age could be imbalanced between the groups and could therefore bias the estimated treatment effect. To prevent this distortion, let's divide the eighty participants by age, splitting them into groups of forty old people and forty young people, with each age group in its own separate table (table 2.3).

Notice that the old people were sicker more often than the young people: $25/40 = 62.5$ percent of the time versus $15/40 = 37.5$ percent of the time. Now when I look among the old people, I see that risk of severe illness in the vaccinated group is $15/25 = 60$ percent. The risk of severe illness in the unvaccinated group of old people is $10/15 = 67$ percent. Therefore, my risk difference is 60 percent − 67 percent = −7 percent. I would conclude that vaccination helps prevent severe illness in older people. Checking the same numbers for young people, I find the risks to be $5/15 = 33$ percent and

TABLE 2.3

Occurrence of severe illness in relation to COVID-19 vaccination status, stratified by age

Old	Vaccination	No vaccination	Total
Sick	15	10	25
Not sick	10	5	15
Total	25	15	40

Young	Vaccination	No vaccination	Total
Sick	5	10	15
Not sick	10	15	25
Total	15	25	40

10/25 = 40 percent, so that the risk difference is 33 percent − 40 percent = −7 percent. So, I would conclude that the vaccination also helps prevent serious illness in younger people. Each stratum of the dataset has the same number of people, so I can take the simple average of −7 percent and −7 percent and conclude that the overall effect here is really −7 percent, a value that is different from my unadjusted ("crude") estimate of 0 percent difference.

Why did the stratified analysis give me a different answer? It is because the crude estimate was *confounded* by age. Age was associated with vaccination (62.5 percent of old people were vaccinated compared to 37.5 percent of young people), and age was predictive of severe illness (62.5 percent versus 37.5 percent). So the crude risk difference was a mix of the two effects: the effect of age on illness and the effect of vaccine on illness.[10] To unmix these two effects, we stratified by age, estimated the two age-specific effects, and then recombined them. There are other ways to conduct adjustments, for example, by weighting and with regression models, but the conceptual logic is similar. We always worry about confounding in observational data when we have the same sort of triangle of factors as in the example above (figure 2.1).

We generally don't worry about confounding in a well-conducted randomized trial because in that design people are not allowed to select their own treatments. Instead, the investigator flips a coin and assigns the treatment based only on that randomization. This balances all other variables, as we saw in the previous coin–flipping game. From figure 2.1, it is easy to see that the confusion arises in observational data because age is both a cause of vaccination and a cause of severe illness. In a randomized trial, however, the only cause of receiving the treatment is the coin flip, and we are confident that coin flips cannot cause severe illness. In a study in which all vaccinations are determined by coin flips, we expect the average age in the vaccinated group to be approximately equal to the average age in the unvaccinated group.[11]

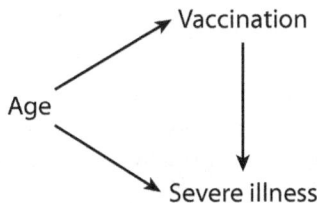

Figure 2.1 Structural relationship between age, vaccination status, and severe illness.

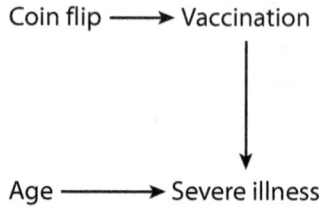

Coin flip ⟶ Vaccination

Age ⟶ Severe illness

Figure 2.2 Structural relationship between age, vaccination status, and severe illness in a randomized trial.

This is represented in the diagram in figure 2.2 by the absence of any arrow connecting age to vaccination status. Severe illness can have many causes besides age. Perhaps there are genetic or behavioral factors that pre-dispose to one suffering a more severe case of COVID-19. We don't need to know about all these other causes because our interest is in the effect of vac-cination, and none of these other causes of severe illness are associated in any way with randomly assigned vaccination. One can think of confounding as an imbalance of any of these variables that can cause the outcome across the treatment groups. There is no such imbalance expected in the randomized trial because vaccination is set by coin flips and only by coin flips. In obser-vational studies, however, statistical adjustments for confounding are methods to balance the covariates across the levels of treatment, in the same way that they would be balanced by random assignment of the treatment in a trial.

This book focuses on racial and ethnic disparities. This is a setting in which confounding problems can be somewhat more subtle and confusing but also more ubiquitous because race and ethnicity are predictive of so many factors that are relevant for outcomes of interest. Take for example the longstanding question of racial differences in IQ scores in the United States, a topic that has generated an enormous and contentious literature.[12] Is it possible to imagine any covariate that would be relevant for IQ score that would *not* be imbalanced across racial or ethnic groups? Nutrition, exposure to lead in one's environment, early life stimulation, education—one would never run out of things to adjust for, and one would never know if some other important cause of IQ was missed.

The randomized trial is considered the gold standard for causal attribution because it balances all other factors between the treated and untreated groups. It would seem that race and ethnicity could never be assigned purposefully by an investigator, so how could we apply this logic when the focus of the study is on race as the treatment? Interestingly, sex is quite different from race in this regard because sex is essentially assigned randomly to all individuals at conception.[13] To appreciate this distinction, notice that the effect of race is confounded by the race of one's parents in a way that the effect of sex is not.[14] Indeed, this distinction has been offered as one explanation for why, under modern progressive social conventions, people may transition from one gender to another but not from one racial identity to another.[15]

But as we discussed in chapter 1, race is not necessarily fixed throughout the lifetime of an individual. Even so, it seems implausible that it could ever be assigned by fiat in the context of an experimental trial. Therefore, we must reason carefully about the effects of race, even without the capacity to assign it to people by flipping a coin. To accomplish this, we can consider the idea of a *counterfactual*. A counterfactual is a hypothetical alternate condition that differs from the one we observe in our world. Historians frequently engage in counterfactual speculations. What might have happened if Abraham Lincoln had survived his assassination in 1865? What if Adolph Hitler hadn't survived the plot to assassinate him in 1944?[16] In causal inference, it can be useful to think of counterfactual outcomes for treated and untreated individuals had they received the alternative condition. Any difference between those two values would constitute an individual causal effect, and the value we estimate in a study is just the average of all the individual causal effects in the study population.

In the case of a racial category as the treatment of interest in some social context, for example being Black versus white, this line of thinking suggests that we would need to compare the treatment of a white person to what would have happened to that same person if, counterfactually, they were perceived to be a Black person. This naturally raises important questions about what it means to be "the same person" with a different race and how such a transition might be accomplished realistically. The first concrete example of this kind of counterfactual racial experiment of which I am aware is the 1961 best-selling book *Black Like Me* by journalist John Howard Griffin. The author underwent treatment by a dermatologist to turn his skin dark so that he was perceived by others to be Black.[17] He then documented his experiences traveling through the American South. As a way of eliciting and comparing social treatment for the same person as Black and as white, this sort of crossover design is intriguing and, assuming that the social perception is convincing, holds all other covariates constant to isolate the effect of race or at least the social perception of race.

Clever social scientists have seized on this idea to make randomized race assignments for quantifying the effect of perceived race on a decision-maker's judgment. In a pioneering example of this approach in 1988, sociologists Marti Loring and Brian Powell wrote down a description of a fictional psychiatric case that was intended to represent undifferentiated mental illness. They labeled this written description randomly with one of four possible race/sex designations (Black or white, male or female) or to a fifth condition lacking demographic information.[18] The profiles were then presented to a large number of psychiatrists by mail, and they were asked to form a diagnosis and return this to the investigators. Even though the case vignette text was identical, the resulting diagnoses varied substantially by the race and sex of the patients. For example, the psychiatrists were more likely to diagnose the Black men with paranoid schizophrenia. Those given no race or sex designations were most likely to avoid diagnosis entirely—the psychiatrists claimed the case was too ambiguous to form a diagnosis. Because of the random assignment of race and sex, there could be no confounding. That means that we can interpret these differences as the causal effects of race and sex. Crucially, however, these are not the effects of race and sex located in the bodies of participants, who aren't real people, but rather the effects of race and sex residing in the minds of the psychiatrists.

Many other fields have exploited similar designs, especially in economics, where they are referred to collectively as "audit studies."[19] For example, Marianne Bertrand and Sendhil Mullainathan sent fictional resumes to help-wanted ads in Boston and Chicago newspapers, randomly assigning names that "sounded" like they belonged alternatively to Black applicants or white applicants—Lakisha and Jamal compared to Emily and Greg, for instance. The applications were otherwise identical.[20] The white names received 50 percent more callbacks for interviews. The experimental control, with all factors held common except for the apparent race of the applicant, once again guarantees a convincing counterfactual applicant. There can be no variables, measured or unmeasured, that are correlated with race and independently predictive of the outcome. The psychiatric patients or job applicants in these designs cannot possibly have any hidden characteristics detected by the judges (the psychiatrists or the prospective employers) because they don't even really exist. Any perceived differences between race groups are therefore attributable to the racial stereotypes or prejudices that the judges might hold, which are exactly the effects that the investigators seek to isolate and quantify.

This sort of individually matched crossover design for race has been widely applied, but it also has its critics. One skeptic of this approach is the sociologist of law Issa Kohler-Hausmann, who explained her doubts in a law review article that began with the iconic 1984 *Saturday Night Live* sketch "White Like Me," in which Eddie Murphy inverted this crossover, becoming a white man to experience racial privilege.[21] Kohler-Hausmann is concerned that race modifies the meaning of all the covariates. That is, an investigator might assign the same years of completed education for the Black and white applicants, but the prospective employer examining the two applications might hold the belief that the education received by a typical Black applicant would be different in some qualitative way from the education received by a typical white applicant. If so, they may believe that these candidates do in fact differ in their educational formation, even though the investigator has assigned them an equal number of completed years of schooling. Because Kohler-Hausmann is concerned that all covariates will probably be modified in their interpretation by race of the applicant in this way, she is skeptical that we learn much about racism by studying the swapping of race labels, rather than understanding the larger historical, political, and economic systems that determine the social consequences to these labels. In short, she argues that such studies may miss the forest for the trees.

A somewhat related critique of audit studies had been expressed with greater formality two decades earlier by the economist James Heckman. He pointed out that even if all relevant covariates are measured, other modeling improprieties, such as an incorrect specification of the model form, can lead to bias in causal estimations.[22] If the decision depends on an unmeasured characteristic exceeding some critical threshold value, then changes in the distribution of the unmeasured characteristic can also lead to observed inequality even in the absence of discrimination. Consider a hypothetical study of gender discrimination in tenure decisions for women scientists at elite universities. Suppose that some unmeasured aspect of intellectual ability (IQ) has the same average value of 100 in men and in women but greater variability in men. If the tenure decision rests on some absolute threshold of ability, say 130, then the longer right tail of the distribution of this unmeasured trait in men will give them a higher probability of exceeding this threshold and therefore of getting tenure, even when there is no discrimination and no sex difference in average ability (figure 2.3).[23]

The past president of Harvard, the economist Lawrence Summers, cited this same argument in 2005 in a small seminar in which he was speculating

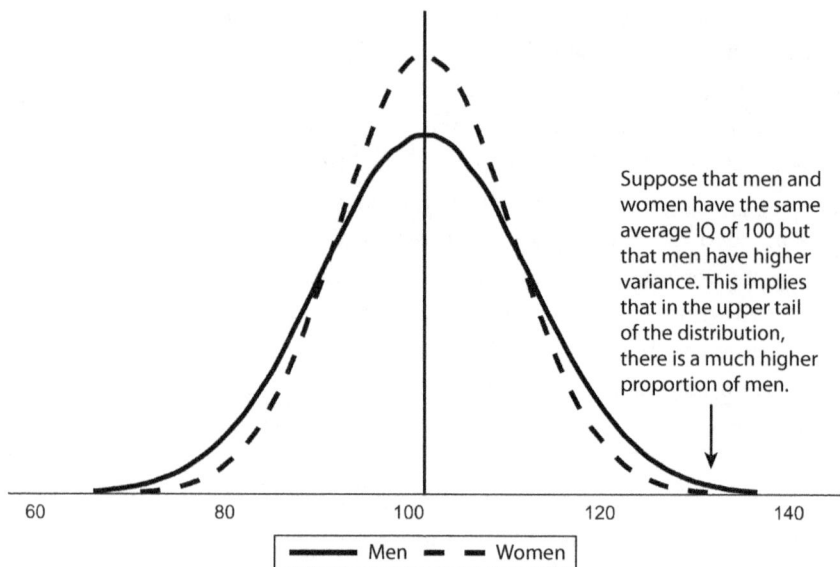

Suppose that men and women have the same average IQ of 100 but that men have higher variance. This implies that in the upper tail of the distribution, there is a much higher proportion of men.

60   80   100   120   140

—— Men — — Women

Figure 2.3 Hypothetical distributions of IQ by gender with equal mean but unequal variance.

on possible explanations for the underrepresentation of women in elite academic settings.[24] Outrage followed, and Summers eventually resigned from his position.

Despite these critiques, audit studies and other counterfactual designs are still used widely in many fields. When the focus is on racial discrimination on the part of a decision-maker, potentially affected by the (perceived) race or ethnicity of the study participant, this same logic can be cautiously extended to the context of real patients rather than imagined ones. For example, Knox Todd, a professor of emergency medicine, and his colleagues considered the causal effect of patient race on receipt of pain medication in a hospital emergency room.[25] They analyzed records from one urban emergency department in Atlanta, selecting for study all self-identified Black and white patients presenting with uncomplicated long-bone fractures over several years. They collected all available medical and demographic information on the patients along with the quantity of pain medication administered to them. Then they used statistical modeling to adjust simultaneously for all the variables that could potentially be associated with race and predictive of pain treatment, such as age, education, and comorbidities. For example, if a higher proportion of Black patients were female and if females generally receive more pain medication, then sex could be a confounder of the causal effect.

After adjusting for the measured confounders, the investigators found that white patients were much more likely to receive pain medication than Black patients, even though they had similar complaints of pain documented in their medical records. The risk of receiving no pain medication at all was 66 percent greater for Black patients, an effect that could not be explained by any confounding factor known to the investigators. Unlike the experiments of authors like Loring and Powell, in which patients are completely imaginary, these emergency room studies of pain medication involved real patients, with both measured and unmeasured characteristics. Of course, the race of the study subjects could not be randomly assigned, and so one can reasonably doubt whether a Black patient with similar measured indicators really forms a convincing counterfactual for that same patient had they been white. There is always the possibility of some important confounder being unmeasured, such as some legitimate counterindication for pain medications like an allergy, if this unmeasured factor happens to be more or less common across race groups.

The reason why I consider this pain medication study to be convincing, however, is because the authors are emergency room physicians who routinely make decisions about dispensing pain medication. If there were some important clinical factor for making a decision about pain medication, wouldn't these authors be exactly the people who would know about this factor? The authors could not think of any legitimate reason beyond the variables measured why anyone should get more or less pain medication than someone else presenting with the same complaints. Without any legitimate explanation for the gap, they were left with only one explanation: racial discrimination. That is to say, the (irrational) influence of a patient's race on the decision-making of the doctor. There are many similar studies employing this basic design, such as a paper by anesthesiologists examining the racial disparity in prophylactic treatment for anesthesia-induced nausea.[26] Once again, the clinician authors know all the plausible indications for treatment, so they can exhaust the legitimate reasons why groups would be treated differently, leaving only the illegitimate reasons. Or, for a nonmedical example, consider the role of covariates in explaining racial disparities in approving applicants for bank loans. Black applicants are denied mortgage loans twice as often as white applicants in the United States. This looks like the same kind of overt discrimination, but bankers argue that differential approval reflects objective differences in creditworthiness as indicated by factors such as debt-to-income levels. Using a dataset of almost nine million loan applications submitted from 2018 to 2019, economists at the Federal Reserve Board recently found that 17 percent of Black applicants were refused, compared with 8 percent of white applicants. Accounting for available creditworthiness variables and remaining blinded to applicant race, this disparity reduced to less than two percentage points in adjusted analyses.[27] Of course the disadvantaged material conditions of the applicants still reflect a long history of structural racism, but the adjusted analysis somewhat exonerates the loan officers from the kind of racially biased decision-making evident in Knox Todd's emergency room studies.

Bear in mind that these are studies of treatment decisions and are therefore entirely different from studies with an interest in identifying the causal effects of race inside the body of a patient rather than inside the mind of a doctor or a banker. Consider instead a study of race as a cause of hypertension in Black versus white patients (discussed in chapter 11). In that setting, one can no longer be confident of the absence of unmeasured confounders because we do not know all the causes of hypertension or even most of them. Therefore, observational studies of race effects on disease etiology do not provide convincing counterfactuals in the way that studies of race effects on decision-making do. This is a key distinction.[28]

Moreover, notice that there is a very different implication when race is the focus of the study versus when race is merely a covariate that might confound another treatment. This is because for the variable that is the treatment, we must necessarily invoke the analogy of a laboratory experiment in which one can assign this quantity randomly. To take the estimate as an unbiased causal effect in the earlier example about vaccination for COVID-19, we had to believe that vaccination was uncorrelated with all other causes of the outcome. This is exactly what would be achieved if vaccination were randomly assigned. This assumption was violated by age, which was a cause of both vaccination and severe illness. Therefore, we had to stratify by age and then assume that, within each age stratum, vaccination was as good as randomly assigned, meaning it was not correlated with any other causes of the outcome. This is the same as if we conducted one randomized assignment of vaccination among young people and another randomized assignment of vaccination among older people. Even so, we never needed to make any particular assumptions about age; it can be correlated with anything, and it surely is.

Vaccination

Race

Severe illness

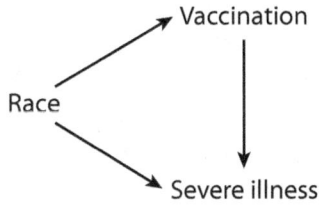

Figure 2.4 Structural relationship between race, vaccination status, and severe illness.

So imagine now that our interest is in the effect of vaccination, which is confounded by race, as shown in figure 2.4. In this case, we would stratify the analysis by race categories to get a valid estimate for the causal effect of vaccination while not being troubled by any difficult philosophical questions about how we might assign race in an experiment. This is because we do not need to imagine any assignment of race in this setting, only a stratification, so that we examine the effect of vaccination on severe illness in one racial group at a time.[29] If the effects were similar across racial groups, we could then recombine these strata again and provide a race-adjusted estimate. Alternatively, if the magnitude of the vaccination effect was very different from one racial group to the next, it might be more informative to keep these categories distinct and present a race-stratified result. There are many legitimate reasons why effects of a treatment like vaccination could truly be heterogeneous across strata of race or ethnicity. For example, if infection rates or risks of severe illness among the infected are much higher in one group compared to another, then the impact of vaccination can also be much higher in that group. This is the logic of targeting influenza vaccination to the elderly, for example, because we expect vaccination to prevent more deaths among that higher-risk subpopulation.[30]

Finally, I should note that not everyone is hung up by the ambiguity surrounding a causal effect of race or ethnicity because of the conceptual problem of assigning these in a hypothetical experiment. We can clearly study the effect of racial discrimination in an experimental setting by controlling what information is presented to the "judge." But what about the effect of race itself, in the body of a person instead of in the mind of the judge? Some scholars are dogmatic about the hypothetical treatment assignment mechanism, arguing that the *way* you make the assignment can change the effect, and therefore, you can't estimate a causal effect unless you specify that mechanism of assignment. For example, what is the effect of obesity on heart disease? Many scholars object that this question is hopelessly ambiguous because there are so many ways to intervene on obesity—by assigning someone to eat less, exercise more, and so on. These different interventions could have distinct effects on heart disease, and therefore, without being more specific about which intervention is intended, one can't claim to quantify any specific causal effect.[31] By this same logic, one could not seek to estimate an unconfounded causal effect of race or ethnicity on any outcome without some explanation for how these characteristics would be assigned.[32]

Other thinkers find this objection ridiculous. They are content to engage in thought experiments involving contrasts of racial identity even if there is no way to accomplish these changes of identity in the real world.[33] After all, they would argue, one can state that the moon causes the tides and even quantify that effect with great precision, all the while having no proposed strategy for getting rid of the moon. There is therefore no barrier to causal inference just because the race or ethnicity of an individual can't be experimentally manipulated, they argue. And there is yet another school of thought that argues that race and ethnicity are in fact highly manipulable because race and ethnicity are social conventions, constantly modified by policies, court decisions, and social movements.[34] For example, the civil rights movement changed what "Black" meant, socially and materially, in the United States, just as World War II internment policies changed the implications of what it meant to be ethnically Japanese.

These conceptual and philosophical debates rage on in the literature and will not soon be resolved. In the meantime, we must make progress studying racial and ethnic disparities, using the tools of statistical analysis as best we can, while staying vigilant about their shortcomings. Some analytic decisions, like adjustment for covariates, might hinge on which perspective the authors embrace, and so it may often be necessary for them to articulate a position about their preferred conceptual framework. Simple causal diagrams like we saw in this chapter are useful in explaining to the reader how treatment is viewed in relation to covariates that are accounted for in the analysis, and these diagrams can also represent other structural problems discussed later, such as selection bias. There may not be a right approach or a wrong approach with respect to these causal debates. But all the same, it's best for an investigator to pick a framework and make that choice clear so that readers understand the analytic decisions that follow.

CHAPTER III

Making Other Worlds

T
he previous chapter explained causal inference as the attempt to estimate what would happen to an individual or a population if they were (perhaps hypothetically) treated one way versus another way. Epidemiologists might be interested in illness as a consequence of taking a drug versus taking a placebo, whereas economists might be interested in wages as a function of workers receiving job training or not. Ideally, we would actually perform a true experiment in which we assigned comparable people to these options and observed what happened. Most of the time, however, real experiments of this kind are impractical. For example, we could not set up experiments to measure outcomes that occur decades later, as in the case of smoking and lung cancer. Or they are unethical. We can't force potentially deleterious conditions on people. Or they are simply impossible. There is just no practical way to compel people to be lifelong smokers, or to be obese, or to receive high versus low levels of education.

In all these settings in which experiments are not realistic options, scientists rely on observational data, which are the recorded experiences of factually treated and untreated people who freely happened upon those treatments through circumstances outside the control of investigators. In these settings, the threat of confounding generally looms large. If there is any reason why a person was treated that also happens to be predictive of the outcome, then the observed association will not have a causal interpretation. The crude data must therefore be subjected to statistical manipulations to intentionally distort the raw observations. We do this to reduce or eliminate biases so that the numbers can be interpreted causally. But we must pay careful attention to what exactly we are doing to the data and the ramifications of these purposeful distortions.

Recall the previous example of an observational study of vaccination for COVID-19 and severe illness. In that example, we were concerned that the treated group was, on average, older than the untreated group. Age is a *nuisance* to us in this scenario. It contaminates the observed vaccine effect with illness risk that has nothing to do with vaccination. To solve this problem, we need to remove age variation from the comparison, which can be done by matching, conditioning, or weighting. In matching, we would pair each vaccinated person with a similarly aged unvaccinated person and sum up the outcome differences across these pairs. Similarly, conditioning simply means stratifying on the confounder in the model. That would be like comparing outcomes among sixty-six-year-olds, then among sixty-seven-year-olds, and so on across the entire age range and then averaging over those results. This is essentially what we did in the stratified analysis in chapter 2 when we divided the population into older and younger participants and then combined the stratum-specific associations. If we had enough people, we could do this in finer strata, thus removing even more of the potential bias. Finally, weighting just means taking the age stratum–specific death rates and applying those rates to a new age distribution, a technique that is commonly referred to as "standardization." This weighting technique is a longstanding and simple approach, and so it is used almost universally to address differential age structure of populations when reporting population surveillance of mortality. For example, numbers appearing in reports from the U.S. Centers for Disease Control and Prevention (CDC) and other government agencies are all generally age adjusted as a routine procedure. They do this to combat potential confounding because age is the most important predictor of mortality and many other outcomes. So if two groups are compared and one is older on average than the other, the contrast of crude rates is potentially misleading, just as it was in our chapter 2 example.

Consider this next example comparing mortality rates in 2015–2016 for Maine, Utah, and the entire United States (table 3.1). The rate is just the number of deaths in a year divided by the number of people at risk of dying in that year. Looking at the last row of the table, one can observe that Maine has a death rate of 1,077 people per 100,000 residents, whereas Utah's death rate is 583 people per 100,000 residents per year. That is to say, Utah's death

TABLE 3.1

Average annual deaths and mortality rates per 100,000 population, 2015–2016

Ages	Maine			Utah			United States		
	Deaths	Population	Rate	Deaths	Population	Rate	Deaths	Population	Rate
0–14	107	208,282	51	382	770,450	50	32,770	60,995,928	54
15–34	327	314,083	104	871	932,272	93	86,101	88,086,844	98
35–54	1,097	344,703	318	1,765	716,105	246	249,445	83,517,390	299
55–74	4,303	358,587	1,200	5,021	474,033	1,059	865,663	69,260,905	1,250
75+	8,497	104,812	8,106	9,586	128,066	7,485	1,494,323	20,412,100	7,321
Total	14,330	1,330,466	1,077	17,623	3,020,925	583	2,728,302	322,273,167	847

Source: Centers for Disease Control and Prevention, National Center for Health Statistics. National Vital Statistics System, Mortality: Compressed Mortality File 1999–2016 on CDC WONDER Online Database, released June 2017. Data are from the Compressed Mortality File 1999–2016 Series 20 No. 2U, 2016, as compiled from data provided by the fifty-seven vital statistics jurisdictions through the Vital Statistics Cooperative Program. Accessed at http://wonder.cdc.gov/cmf-icd10.html on November 28, 2022.

rate is roughly half as large as Maine's. This is an astounding difference and might lead to all manner of speculation about the health benefits of Mormonism or downhill skiing. But this is simply not a fair comparison because the populations differ dramatically in age structure—Maine is much older. The population column reveals that almost 8 percent of Maine's residents are seventy-five years old or older compared to only about 4 percent of Utah residents. If I'm in the mortuary business and I need to know how many caskets I will need, the crude number is the better one for me to pay attention to. But if I am interested in life expectancy and want to compare states to see which one offers its citizens the longer average experience on Earth, I need to adjust for age structure to make the comparison more fair. I can do that by standardization, which applies the age category–specific rates from each state to a common (or "standard") population denominator. We are free to choose any standard population we want. It could be either state, for example, or the combination of the two states, or an external standard like the entire U.S. population. We'll use that last one, the age distribution of the entire United States.

The rate in the youngest age group in Maine is 51, so we multiply this by the U.S. population in that age group, which is nearly 61 million. We do the same in the next row, moving down the age categories and summing up all these products before finally dividing by the total U.S. population.[1] This gives us a result of 892 deaths per 100,000 Maine residents per year. This number is not the real death rate in Maine but rather is the rate of death that *would be* observed if Maine had the same population age structure as the rest of the country. Now we do the same for Utah, starting with the youngest age group and multiplying each age-specific rate in Utah with the denominator population in the entire United States, summing these products, and dividing by the U.S. population. That yields a final value of 800 deaths per 100,000 people per year.[2] These two age-adjusted mortality rates give a very different impression of the disparity between the two states. Maine's crude mortality rate was almost twice as large as Utah's, but its age-adjusted rate is only slightly larger—about 900 in Maine and 800 in Utah—and neither Utah nor Maine is very different from the United States as a whole, which has 847 deaths per 100,000 people per year. Many more people actually die in Maine, but that is mostly because they are older. In fact, the more finely age-adjusted death rates will be even closer together, but I used a small number of age categories to keep things simple for this example. Stratification by narrower age categories better controls for confounding and therefore yields age-adjusted rates that are even more comparable to one another than the ones I have shown here.[3]

Although this calculation is quite simple and routine, it's important to bear in mind that we are no longer observing the true difference between groups in the real world but instead the imagined difference in a hypothetical world. All numbers provided in governmental and scientific reports are subjected to this kind of intentional distortion. We rarely focus on the true numbers of deaths. Because we use age-adjusted numbers almost exclusively, we sometimes forget that we do not live in this imaginary world and that the adjusted numbers do not describe what is really happening in our unadjusted real world. Nonetheless, the comparison made in this imaginary world has its advantages. In the case of comparing Maine and Utah, age adjustment provides a better sense of the relative success of each state at keeping its citizens alive. In the example of evaluating the effects of a treatment effect like taking a COVID-19 vaccine, the adjusted rates may be better at predicting the outcome of some future action in our world, such as taking the vaccine or not.

But many things can go wrong in generating this model of an imaginary world. First, we have to pick the imaginary world out of an unlimited set of possibilities because any set of weights can serve as the age standard. We also rely on other assumptions, some of which could be mistaken. How can we check that the adjusted estimate is really better than the unadjusted estimate? The most secure answer is to conduct a randomized trial, so that an investigator flips a coin to assign the treatment, such as vaccination, for each person in the study. Under this design, if the sample size is large, we do not expect any important imbalances in factors such as age between treatment groups. Therefore, association can be safely interpreted as causation. Things can still go wrong in the context of the randomized study, like people dropping out or refusing their assignments. But these can all be checked and adjusted for if necessary. But checking modeled results with a randomized trial is often impractical or unethical. For example, statistical models comparing smokers and nonsmokers in the 1950s suggested that smoking was a cause of lung cancer. It was determined that there was no ethical design by which humans could be compelled to smoke or not smoke by random assignment, and so this verification was never attempted. Nonetheless, based on many other pieces of evidence, including adjusted estimates from observational studies and experimental studies in animals, it was concluded that the observed association between smoking and lung cancer was indeed causal.

Many other models similarly cannot be checked against randomized trials, such as how mortality risk differs between Maine and Utah. Let's return to the main theme of this book, racial and ethnic comparisons. It is clear that these demographic traits cannot be assigned in trials, although there are several clever designs that accomplish something similar, as described in the previous chapter. So, then, what is the criterion for determining better or worse estimation when racial groups are compared in adjusted models? Clearly, the motivation for adjustment may still exist. For example, just as people receiving the COVID-19 vaccine could be older or younger than those who do not, there could be age-distribution differences between racial or ethnic groups that confound their comparison, motivating a model of an imaginary world in which groups have similar age structures that could be directly compared. But if one decides to adjust for age, does one stop there? What other factors beyond age must also be controlled to generate a "fair" comparison? That question is taken up more fully in the next chapter.

The discussion above might seem a bit esoteric, and you might wonder how much it matters that adjusted rates are a fiction. First, it is worth noting that such adjustments can change the data dramatically. Consider a recent evaluation of public health policies in relation to COVID-19 infections and deaths that was conducted by the Institute for Health Metrics and Evaluation (IHME).[4] The authors wanted to compare the pandemic experiences of the fifty states and the District of Columbia, but they recognized that the crude death rates would make for an unfair comparison. Different states had different age and comorbidity distributions that produced different risks for COVID-19 mortality. Therefore, they standardized for the age distribution and prevalence of seven health conditions, using the whole United States as the standard population. They then presented both the crude and adjusted results for comparison.

In the real world of the crude data, West Virginia had the highest COVID-19 mortality—ranked fifty-first out of fifty-one. COVID-19 killed 575 out of every 100,000 residents through July 31, 2022. But West Virginia is a very old and sick state. The authors were more interested in what the COVID-19 mortality experience would have been if West Virginia had the age and health status of the entire United States. Adjusting the age of West Virginians to the average age in the United States, the rate came down from 575 to 478 per 100,000. Adjusting the comorbidity rate took it down from 478 to 322 per 100,000. This, surprisingly, left West Virginia with one of the best pandemic performances in the country—fourteenth out of fifty-one.

51 West Virginia, 51 ●   ● Washington, DC, 50

46   ● Colorado, 47
                                                     ● Idaho, 46
                                                     ● Utah, 45

41   ● Alaska, 42
        Michigan, 40 ●
        Florida, 38 ●
36   Ohio, 36 ●   ● California, 36

31

26

21   Idaho, 21 ●

16   ● Michigan, 16
        Washington, DC, 15 ●   ● West Virginia, 14
        Colorado, 13 ●   ● Florida, 12
11   California, 12 ●

        Alaska, 8 ●   ● Ohio, 8
6

        Utah, 3 ●
1

Rank among states (1 = lowest mortality rate)

Crude death rate rank   Standardized death rate rank

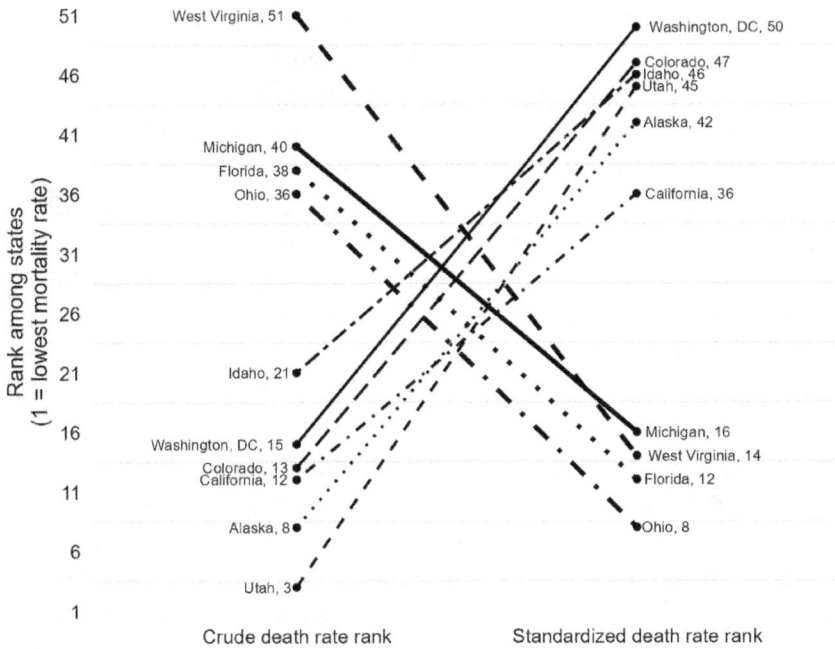

Figure 3.1 How standardization changed state ranks for ten selected states.

Many other states moved in the opposite direction (figure 3.1). Utah, for example, had a crude mortality of 219 per 100,000, in third place out of fifty-one. But accounting for its favorable age and health profile left it with an adjusted mortality of 467 per 100,000. That put Utah in forty-fifth place.

Let's return to the main theme of this book. Here are two real-life examples of adjustment decisions that were consequential for public debates about racial and ethnic disparities. To keep things simple and familiar, we'll stick with age adjustments. The first example involves the choice of the standard for federal health and demographic statistics. For many years, the age distribution found in the 1940 census was used for all federal statistics in the United States. Some statistical reports eventually transitioned to the 1970 census, but this switch wasn't consistent across government agencies.[5] Finally, in the late 1990s, it became clear that a new and uniform standard was needed. The 1940 population was hopelessly out of date. Even the 1970 standard was becoming awkward by the end of the twentieth century, as the population had become older, on average. In 1970, the median age was twenty-eight; by 2000, it was thirty-five. Because of this, federal agencies planned to convert all federal reporting uniformly to the year 2000 age distribution as soon as the new census numbers became available.[6] This change had profound—albeit artefactual—implications for the reporting of racial and ethnic health disparities by the U.S. government.

The underlying problem with how changing the age standard affects reporting of racial and ethnic disparities is a mathematical one, which will be examined in greater detail in chapter 9. For now, the crucial point for this example is that disparities tend to be reported on the *ratio scale*, meaning that they are expressed as the rate in the disadvantaged group divided by the rate in the advantaged group. For example, the year 2020 age-standardized mortality rate in Native Americans and Pacific Islanders was 1,008 per 100,000 people per year. The adjusted rate in non-Hispanic whites was 831 per 100,000 people per year. So the disparity on the ratio scale is called a "relative rate" and is equal to 1,008 divided by 831, which equals 1.21.[7] This number tells us simply that the age-adjusted mortality rate among Native Americans and Pacific Islanders was 21 percent higher than among non-Hispanic whites in 2020. The mathematical problem is that the higher the denominator rate (the bottom number in the fraction), the smaller the ratio tends to be.[8] Because of this relationship between the disparity and the size of the number in the comparator population, relative health disparities tend to be more modest for older people than for younger people because the denominator rates are much higher for older people.

Take the example of cardiovascular disease mortality by race and age group in 2020 (figure 3.2).[9] For men between the ages of thirty-five and forty-four, the rate per 100,000 per year was 103.1 for Black Americans and 43.3 for white Americans. That's a disparity of 2.38. At ages forty-five to fifty-four, the rates were 297.8 and 135.1, or a disparity of 2.07. You can see that as the rates increase, the ratio disparity decreases. At ages fifty-five to sixty-four, this is 648.9/343.0 = 1.89. At ages sixty-five to seventy-four, it's 1240.1/677.0 = 1.83. And at ages seventy-five to eighty-four, it's 2296.5/1676.4 = 1.37.

The consistent pattern we observe is that older people with higher rates of experiencing the outcome have smaller disparities on the ratio scale. This is just a mathematical artefact of the scale of contrast that is used. For example, the age pattern would be completely opposite if we generated the contrast by subtracting and creating differences instead of dividing and creating ratios (figure 3.3).

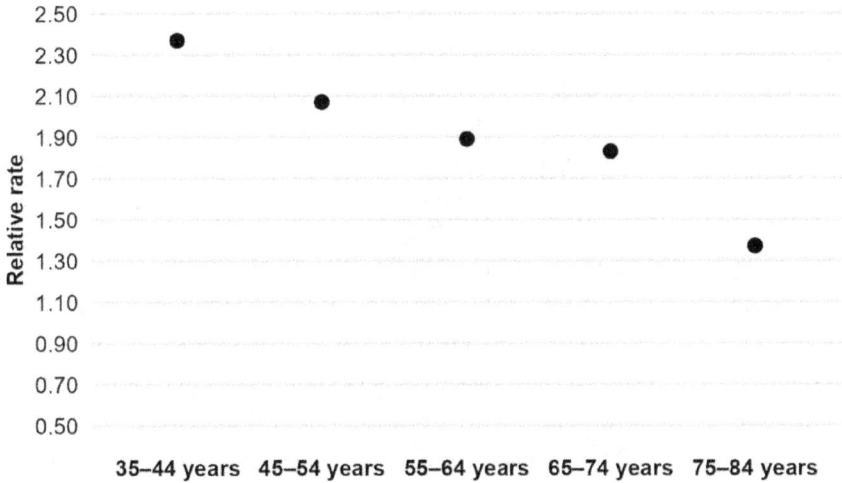

Figure 3.2 Relative rate by race (Black/white) by age: Cardiovascular mortality among men in 2020, United States.

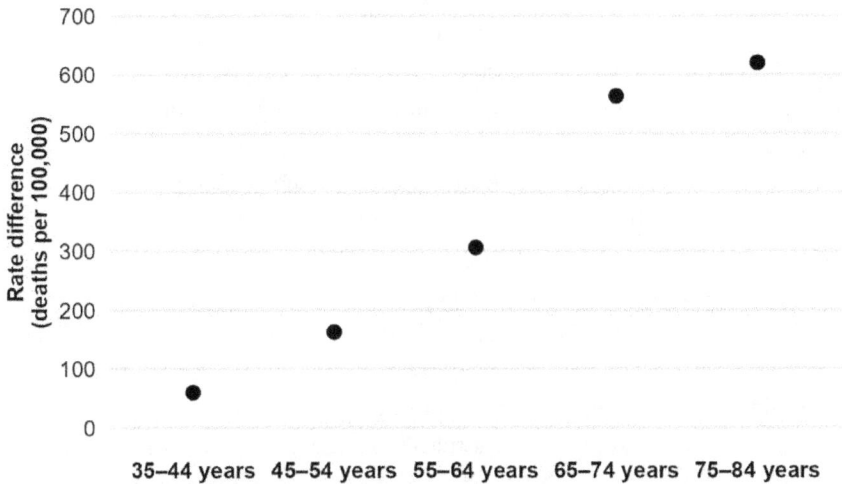

Figure 3.3 Rate difference by race (Black−white) by age: Cardiovascular mortality among men in 2020, United States.

But, for whatever reason, surveillance of disparities by the government is almost always reported on the ratio scale. Therefore, when the age standard is changed to an older distribution, as it was when moving from the 1940 age structures to the 1970 age structures and finally to the year 2000 age structures, the ratio disparities inevitably decrease.

To illustrate the implications of this administrative transition for reported disparities, the epidemiologists Nancy Krieger and David Williams compared the effects of defining the standard population according to the age distributions found in the 1940, 1970, and 2000 U.S. censuses.[10] They considered race and socioeconomic comparisons and documented that the disparities were often dramatically reduced by the change of standard population. Comparing the poorest Hispanics to the richest Hispanics above age forty-five in 1995, for example, the proportion in worse health was five times higher using the 1940 standard but only 3.5 times higher using the year 2000 standard. Thus, about a third of the disparity was magically wiped away by the arbitrary change in standard. Likewise, in non–Hispanic Blacks, this disparity was more than fivefold using the 1940 standard but decreased to a little more than fourfold using the standard from the year 2000. Krieger and Williams found the reported health gap was reduced substantially across all the populations they looked at, often by roughly 20 to 30 percent. And yet no human being was actually better off despite these apparent improvements. These artefactual reductions to health disparities occurred instantaneously when one capricious standard was replaced by another. America suddenly became much less racially unequal in its health profile—at least according to its official statistics. Government exercises a crucial role in monitoring disparities to gauge progress in programs designed to achieve equity, and the administration of President George W. Bush scored a big victory with this obscure policy transition, shaving off a sizable fraction of inequality within months of taking office.

The Krieger and Williams paper is not the only analysis to highlight artefactual changes that arise from differing population age standards. For example, a study of austerity policies in Spain in 2018 mistakenly compared inequalities across a similar administrative change in standard populations and had to be retracted.[11] Another more recent example of how age standardization can become the central issue in a public debate occurred in 2022, when the *New York Times* columnist David Leonhardt published a short online report on the evolution of racial disparities in COVID-19 mortality in that year.[12] Leonhardt noted that over the previous two years, while the pandemic raged in the United States, the per capita death rate from COVID-19 for Blacks was roughly twice as high as it was for whites and Asians. By 2022, however, this disparity disappeared. In fact, it reversed, which he attributed to differential uptake of vaccines. Leonhardt presented a graph of CDC data through the end of May 2022, first in crude numbers and then separately for ages eighteen to forty-nine years and ages sixty-five and older. The data showed how mortality had previously been highest for Blacks in 2020 and 2021 but that, by 2022, it had become highest in whites. "The main culprit is politics," he concluded, noting that only 60 percent of Republicans had been vaccinated compared with 90 percent of Democrats and that Republicans tended to be older and whiter.

This was a simple observation, supported by CDC data, and so might be expected to attract little critical attention. But instead it unleashed a torrent of online protest. An epidemiology blogger named Katelyn Jetelina posted immediately to declare that Leonhardt was "wrong" and that his column constituted "misinformation."[13] An online mob quickly assembled to express the same complaint with more vitriol. Leonhardt, they claimed, had erred by presenting crude rather than age-standardized mortality. "We need to take into account age," wrote Jetelina. "White Americans are far more likely to outlive Black Americans. . . . This is important because age is the strongest risk factor, by far, for dying of COVID." The experts lined up on Twitter behind the crude rates as misinformation and characterized Leonhardt as an ignorant hack who should be fired.[14]

Leonhardt, for his part, tried to respond gently on Twitter to this critique.[15] He acknowledged that age standardization might be another appropriate way of looking at these data, but he insisted that the basic story he told was accurate: Black Americans had died at a higher rate than white Americans earlier in the pandemic, but this pattern had reversed in 2022. Clearly, the crude data reported by Leonhardt are indeed the numbers that pertain to the real world in which we all live, and he had even taken the extra step of stratifying into older and younger age groups out of the same concern, even if he did not take the more abstract journey into a counterfactual world of fully age-standardized rates. Nonetheless, his critics simply did not accept that these numbers of deaths from the real world represented accurate reporting. What they wanted instead were numbers that reflected the rates that would, hypothetically, be observed in an imaginary world in which Black and white Americans had the same age structure. Leonhardt was wrong, wrote epidemiologist Gregg Gonsalves. "Have the common decency to say it. Your analysis was flawed. People have pointed it out and it's a first-year public health student mistake."[16]

Age adjustments are indeed reflexive in almost all epidemiologic surveillance, and all federal statistics are now provided with age standardization to the 2000 census. In this sense, Leonhardt's critics expressed a completely normative viewpoint.[17] At the same time, Leonhardt was engaged in journalism, and it seems perverse to describe the real-world numbers as misinformation. But might real-world numbers be less useful in this specific comparison? If one has an interest in racial inequity, which is the more illuminating way of representing the contrast? Gonsalves and the other critics were in the mainstream of standard practice when they asserted that the age-adjusted figures are the ones that they would normally expect to see.

Nonetheless, one can also make several arguments for why the crude rates would be more informative.[18] It is not the case that the crude numbers are wrong and the adjusted numbers are right but rather that they each reveal a different angle on the truth. The argument for the age-standardized mortality comparison is to remove the irrelevant nuisance of age differences between groups and therefore to fairly compare populations as though they had similar ages. This follows from the simple and indisputable fact that age is the most important independent risk factor for COVID-19 mortality. But the advantage of the crude rates is that they represent the numbers of people who actually died rather than the numbers that would have died under imaginary demographic scenarios. And standardization requires picking a standard, which introduces an arbitrary element as demonstrated by the Krieger and Williams article.

Here are two more compelling reasons to be wary of putting all of one's eggs in the basket of an age-standardized comparison. It is true that non-Hispanic Black American life expectancy had been about four years lower than that of non-Hispanic whites before the pandemic. This had increased to about six years lower by the end of 2021.[19] Why is this so? Clearly a long history of differential social treatment by race (i.e., systemic racism) has fueled a persistent mortality rate gap for as long as modern statistics have been collected. Although this has narrowed steadily in recent decades,[20] the initial two years of the COVID-19 pandemic were a huge setback due to a sudden surge in Black mortality. It is therefore clear that COVID-19 was itself a major cause of the discrepant age distributions by the end of 2021.[21] Calculating the age-standardized mortality rates in 2022 using a prepandemic population standard basically says, "Let's assume that COVID-19 did *not* take a differential toll on Black Americans in 2020 and 2021 and then calculate, under that premise, what would be implied about racial disparities in 2022." It is a premise that assumes the opposite of what you're looking for! Suppose I were to pose the following question. Assuming cigarettes did not cause any lung cancer cases in 2020 and 2021, is there an excess of lung cancer among smokers in 2022?[22] Why insist on using age-adjusted rates in the COVID-19 example, when the premise of equal age structures is contradicted by the factual effects of COVID-19 on the age structure difference?

Here is a second and even more persuasive reason to be critical of the age-standardized rates as the single right answer to this question: Why stop with age? The argument for adjusting for age is that it is distributed differently by race and is also independently predictive of mortality. Both of those assumptions are clearly true of age, but they are not true *only* of age. They are also true of many other variables. Consider state of residence, for example. Distribution of population by race is hugely different by state. More than a third of the population of Mississippi is Black; almost no one in Montana is Black.[23] State is also strongly predictive of COVID-19 mortality. At least eight states had cumulative COVID-19 mortality rates above 400 per 100,000 population, including Arizona and Oklahoma. However, there were seven states below 200 per 100,000 population, including Washington and Utah.[24] So if age must be adjusted, then, by that logic, state must also be adjusted. As long as we are leaving the real world and entering into the world of hypothetical models in which age distribution is the same for Blacks and whites, why not also make them live in equal proportions in each state? And why stop there? One could also adjust for health insurance, obesity, income, housing, and dozens and dozens of other racial differences that affect COVID-19 mortality. Not the least of these is vaccination, which is what Leonhardt speculated was the main driver of the flip in rates that he observed. If we are adjusting away the difference in age, why not also the difference in vaccination? The point is that once you enter imaginary worlds, there is no reason to stop halfway. This means that there can't be a single right answer among the adjusted estimates because we can't possibly agree on a single right list of the adjustments to be made or the standard populations from which to draw these adjustments.

There is only one true crude disparity, and that is the disparity we measure in the real world. But there are an infinite number of potential adjusted disparities. Of course, adjustment can also be illuminating, and there are often good reasons to do it. But it is not an issue of right or wrong statistical analysis, as suggested by Leonhardt's critics. Both the crude and the adjusted contrasts can be useful in understanding the nature of the disparity. And this story happens to have an even more astonishing conclusion. In the end, Leonhardt was completely vindicated. Despite all the shoot-from-the-hip accusations of statistical malfeasance when the article appeared, nobody took the time to actually perform the age standardization using real data. Once they did, they found that even in the age-standardized data, the 2022 flip of racial disparities was clearly apparent. Whites unambiguously had the highest age-adjusted COVID-19 mortality rates.[25] Leonhardt himself wrote up this result in a column a few months later, showing that age standardization did not change his earlier story.[26] He again attributed the flip to aggressive vaccination outreach and even offered an olive-branch quote to Jetelina, the blogger who launched the earlier criticism against his first article. "The inequities have largely dissipated in recent weeks and months, even after adjusting for age," she agreed.

Other authors have followed up on this question, including a paper by the public health graduate student Dielle Lundberg and colleagues that focused on the fact that the first year of the pandemic was largely an urban phenomenon and that it increasingly shifted out of cities in 2021 and 2022.[27] Because racial and ethnic groups have very different distributions in the population between metropolitan and nonmetropolitan regions, this presents an important evolution in the population at risk, and it has real implications for disparities. The authors reported that only about 5 percent of COVID-19 deaths had occurred in nonmetropolitan areas during the first wave of the pandemic, but this increased to more than 20 percent of deaths in subsequent waves of the Delta and Omicron strains of coronavirus. The researchers therefore standardized not only for age but also for racial and ethnic differences by metropolitan versus nonmetropolitan residence. In doing so, they discovered that although death rates for non-Hispanic whites had indeed increased relative to other groups, a large portion of this change was accounted for by the increasing penetration of the pandemic into nonmetropolitan areas where a disproportionate share of non-Hispanic white adults reside.

We have seen that observational data can be confounded by an imbalance between treated and untreated groups in other important causes of the outcome. Statisticians have a number of solutions to this problem, including standardization, in which the samples are reweighted to show what the treatment contrast would be in the imaginary world without that imbalance.

Working through a simple example, we have seen how informative such an adjustment can be but also some of the limitations and caveats of adjustments. The choice of the standard for the weights can be somewhat arbitrary, and yet this choice can lead to big changes in the obtained estimates. The adjusted numbers are also a kind of fiction, and they might involve premises that are more or less sensible, depending on the chosen imaginary world. In the COVID-19 example, we could interpret the adjusted estimates as the disparity in mortality that would be observed if we were willing to assume there were no historical disparities in mortality, which seems like an unreasonable or self-contradictory premise. Besides that, age is only one of countless possible variables that are imbalanced between racial and ethnic groups. For example, although racial groups differ in their age structure, they differ even more profoundly in where they live. So how do we select the right covariates so that we can think of what it would mean for a disparity to be sufficiently adjusted? This question is taken up in the next chapter.

CHAPTER IV

Crude Versus Adjusted Racial and Ethnic Comparisons

We have seen that the effect of a treatment estimated from observational data can be *confounded* by another variable, meaning that the other variable is associated with the treatment and is a cause of the outcome. In this circumstance, the two effects—that of the treatment and of the other variable—get mixed together and confused, which is the original meaning of the word *confounded*.[1] When the other variable is measured, there are various statistical adjustments we can use to unconfound the treatment effect so that we might obtain the effect that would have been seen in a randomized trial of the treatment. Remember, a key advantage of a large randomized trial is that all other variables, whether measured or not, are distributed equally between the treated and untreated groups. This is the basic logic behind the common statistical adjustments that occur in most scientific papers in fields like medicine, education, economics, sociology, and psychology.

The situation is a bit different, however, when we consider the examination of racial and ethnic disparities. A large randomized trial is the "gold standard" for studies of treatment effects because in the randomized trial, there are no other unbalanced factors—treated and untreated groups of participants differ only in their receipt of the treatment, not in any other respect. We could not expect this kind of complete similarity for racial and ethnic groups. We might accept, for example, that Mexican Americans can eat more cilantro on average than Black Americans without thinking that this is problematic for most causal hypotheses. Besides, this "treatment" of being classified into one or another demographic category could never be randomly assigned to real people, and so the randomized trial cannot serve as the gold standard of what we hope to accomplish with statistical adjustments. Even if we were to randomize some manipulable intervention to individuals in different racial or ethnic groups, we would not necessarily expect these treatment effects to have to be the same across groups.[2] And yet at the same time, it seems clear that such adjustments may be warranted. Suppose that the groups being compared are Cuban Americans and Mexican Americans and the outcome is cancer, which has a rapidly increasing risk as a person ages. The Cuban American population happens to be older overall than the Mexican American population, and so they naturally have more incident cases of cancer. A common-sense judgment is that this crude rate is an inadequate summary, rooted in the intuitive sense that differences due to age are not germane to the question of ethnic equity in cancer risk.[3]

Because we are not studying a manipulable treatment with the intention of making a policy to encourage or discourage any intervention in the population, we need another basis for adjusting the contrast. Clearly, the focus when using demographic groups like race and ethnicity and even gender is to detect systematic differences between these groups in exposure to the causes of the outcome. If Cuban Americans have a higher cancer rate, even compared to other ethnicities with the same age, then there must be some carcinogenic factor that is more common in this group. This could be important to notice simply as a way of discovering new causes of cancer in every group. More frequently, we conduct such comparisons because groups with excess risk warrant being targeted for prevention or screening because the excess risk is a disparity that we consider unnecessary, unnatural, or unacceptable. The motivation for adjustment is therefore finding groups that have unacceptable disadvantages so that these can be targeted. It is not immediately obvious which differences qualify for that sort of flagging. For example, women live longer than men in every society. Is this a matter of social injustice or a simple and immutable fact of nature?[4]

Because the motivation to compare groups is to assess equity not equality, we need some kind of theory of fairness to distinguish between the two. Equality is just a mathematical statement that makes no normative judgments about what is right or wrong, what should or should not occur, in an ethical sense. To say that older people die at a higher rate than younger people, for example, is a statement about a mathematical inequality in mortality rates, that some number is bigger than some other number. It does not imply that this is good or bad, natural or unnatural, changeable or unchangeable. That most people consider this to be a fact about the natural world and not an injustice is an ethical judgment imposed over that math. It is a statement about equity rather than equality.[5]

A central point of this chapter follows from this distinction between equality and equity. Crude (unadjusted) statistical assessments of disparities between racial and ethnic groups tell us something about equality or inequality in the strictly mathematical sense. This is rarely the motivation for such work, however. More commonly, the analysts examining disparities are concerned about fairness—about differences that represent injustices or that warrant interventions to ameliorate bias, discrimination, or disparate social treatment. It is this focus on equity rather than equality that necessitates statistical adjustments.

We need models that can correspond to equity judgments, and these are typically adjusted models. The adjustment removes from view the play of factors that are irrelevant or immaterial to the underlying question of fairness. Return to the earlier example of cancer disparities between Cuban Americans and Mexican Americans and the sense that Cubans should not be penalized in this assessment simply for being older. Our real interest is whether a Cuban American of some specific age has higher or lower cancer risk than a Mexican American of the same age. The value judgment underlying this discomfort with the crude comparison is that age is an accepted cause of cancer in the biological sense, and this makes it a permissible cause of cancer in an ethical sense. This means that although cancer is a sad event no matter who gets it, we do not consider it an affront to our sense of justice that older people have higher rates of cancer than younger people. All statistical adjustments for the purpose of equity require a value judgment concerning differences that are ethically permissible and those that are ethically impermissible. Statistical adjustment is meant to eliminate such nuisance variables and allow a "fair" comparison with direct implications for social justice.[6]

What constitutes a fair reason for an inequality versus an unfair reason? This is a topic of many books in philosophy and ethics.[7] It has long been a crucial question in economics and has recently come to the foreground in computer science due to concerns of algorithmic bias.[8] Despite ubiquitous statistical adjustments for this purpose in public health, demography, and health services research, however, it remains little discussed in those circles.

Because statistics is taught as a technical specialty, there is generally little attention to these kinds of ethical questions in training programs, and yet we require ethical judgments to know for which variables we must adjust. Another problem is that such judgments will be situational, legitimately differing from one application to another.

Here is a clear example of this kind of situational variation. The U.S. Institute of Medicine (IOM) published a landmark report in 2003 on racial and ethnic disparities in the provision of healthcare.[9] For the purposes of this congressionally mandated report, the authors defined "disparities" as differences in the quality of healthcare received that are not due to "access-related factors or clinical needs, preference, and appropriateness of intervention." Let's unpack this definition. Most importantly, it excuses all differences that might be blamed on factors outside the control of healthcare providers. This is because the authors were focused on discrimination in the delivery of care. If patients faced barriers in getting to the doctor or didn't even want to go to the doctor, this would be a problem, but from the point of view of the IOM, it would be someone else's problem. This definition also assumes a certain amount of mechanistic knowledge about disparities, because it excuses things due to one set of factors but not those due to another set of factors, requiring that we know the whole causal structure of these disparities to make the attributional distinction.

Given that the IOM report was interested in discrimination by healthcare providers, it needed to extract from the observed (crude) disparity any and all contributions from differential access, differential preferences, and differential appropriateness. So if one ethnic group had lower levels of automobile ownership, presenting a barrier to accessing the clinic, that fact is off the table because it is not the fault of clinicians or the health system. If one ethnic group has less trust in the medical system, that is off the table for the same reason. If one ethnic group just doesn't even want a service as much as another for some cultural reason, this is also off the table. Whatever is left after these extractions can be laid at the feet of health systems and clinicians as their problem to confront and solve. The machinery for taking things off the table is statistical adjustment. Therefore, when adjusting the observed differences for covariates, analysts following the logic and motivation of the 2003 IOM report must pick the covariates that represent the access, preference, and appropriateness factors that are considered to be "permissible."[10] All other differences are labeled as "discrimination" and serve as an indictment against the providers and health systems.

From this example, it is clear that covariate adjustment for disparities will always be subjective and situational, depending on the values and focus of the investigators. Because the IOM authors focused on blaming discriminatory providers, they excused all access factors. But some other investigator may be interested in racial and ethnic differences that arise from broader social factors like structural racism, which would then have to include access barriers and thus require adjusting away fewer covariates. In practice, this means that the IOM authors would adjust for a covariate like automobile ownership, making the racial or ethnic contrast into the imaginary one that would be observed if, counter to fact, both compared groups had equal rates of automobile ownership. Another investigator who is interested in structural racism would want to indict differential transportation as one factor to be blamed, not excused, and so the investigators of this second study would *not* adjust away the disparity due to automobile ownership. In this way, the set of variables to be adjusted must reflect something about the scope of things to be blamed versus excused.

Adjustments may exist to partition responsibility guided by who is to be blamed or not blamed, but this can be difficult to navigate in practice. Recall that a second set of factors excused by the IOM researchers was patient preferences. For example, Black patients with early-stage non–small-cell lung cancer have been found to have worse survival than white patients,[11] and yet it was observed that survival is similar across race group among all those who undergo surgery. Further examination revealed that Blacks were less likely to be offered surgery when it was not clearly indicated and, if it was offered, were more likely to decline the surgery. Being offered surgery less often is clearly the fault of the provider and that would obviously be blamed on them by the IOM investigators. But declining the surgery is a matter of patient preference and so would be excused. How can we understand why one racial or ethnic group would prefer not to have a potentially life-saving surgery? Can we really just chalk that up to preference in the way that someone might prefer Pepsi over Coke? Some more nuanced work attempts to unpack these preferences and finds that patients refusing lung cancer surgery complained of poor physician communication and expressed poor expectations of their prognosis after surgery, which might suggest that providers can indeed influence such decisions after all.[12] If patients have less trust in the physician or the medical system to act in their best interests, should this really be excused away as a matter of mere preference?[13]

We have already seen an example in the previous chapter of an adjustment that could be argued either way with respect to age as a potential confounder of racial differences in COVID-19 mortality. The ambiguity in that example arose because age structure in the population reflects differential mortality, for instance in the recent COVID-19 pandemic. So when examining the impact of race on differential COVID-19 mortality, should one use statistical adjustment to excuse the previous impact of race on differential COVID-19 mortality? This is not an easy question to answer, and reasonable people might disagree.[14] Let's see some other examples that reveal how tricky it can be to agree on a list of permissible variables and what this choice might reveal about assumptions and values.

The Urban Institute publishes a continually updated analysis of the National Assessment of Educational Progress (NAEP), a standardized test administered to a nationally representative sample of U.S. students every other year.[15] Test scores are available for reading and math for fourth graders and eighth graders in every U.S. state. The Urban Institute does not focus on the crude scores, however, but instead explains that a "better way to compare and talk about NAEP performance is to use adjusted NAEP scores that account for demographic differences across students in each state. These adjusted scores allow for students to be compared with their demographically similar peers using factors such as race, receipt of special education services, and status as an English language learner. These are factors we know can affect test results, yet they are not shown in [crude] NAEP scores."[16] Policymakers are interested in comparing state scores because they are interested in understanding the impact of state educational policy on student performance. Their argument is that these policy effects cannot be easily understood based on the crude test scores because of the confounding effects of demographic differences between states.

The crude and adjusted performances differ substantially, having a profound impact on the rankings of the states. Looking at eighth grade math scores in 2019, for example, Louisiana actually scored near the very bottom, but its adjusted rank was in the top half of states (figure 4.1). Mississippi likewise tested almost dead last but was adjusted all the way up into the top ten by the statistical model. Texas ranked fourth in the nation after adjustment despite a true performance in the lower half. In the adjusted world, Texas and Louisiana vastly outperformed New Hampshire and Vermont because this analysis makes more relevant comparisons that are balanced on race and

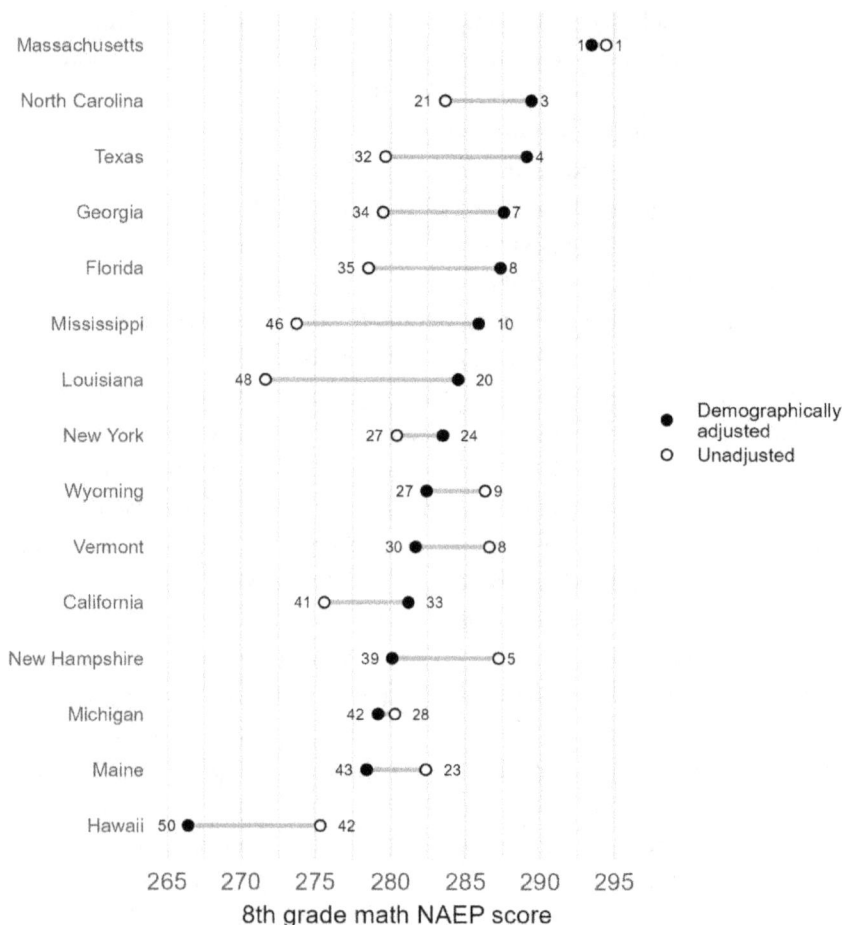

Figure 4.1 Performance on the 2019 National Assessment of Educational Progress (NAEP) for fifteen selected states.

poverty in a way that the real world does not. Just as we did not want to penalize Maine for being older than Utah in the previous example on age standardization, the Urban Institute uses the same sort of statistical adjustments so that Texas will not be punished for having more kids speaking Spanish at home or Louisiana for having more Black children. Given the stated goal of assigning credit or blame to each state's educational policies, this seems reasonable. Each state must educate the students that happen to reside there, whether poor or nonnative English speakers or whatever other demographic characteristic that predicts test scores.

However, to consider a state like Mississippi an educational success story once their demographic challenges are adjusted away, despite objectively testing near the very bottom, one risks normalizing the expectation that poor and minority kids naturally and inevitably perform poorly. One would be hard-pressed to come up with a more striking example of Michael Gerson's "soft bigotry of low expectations" than the casual assertion that a state with low scores is doing perfectly well given the hapless demographic mix of kids that live there.[17] Thus, this adjustment approach treats the ineducability of certain racialized students like a fact of nature to be rendered invisible in the final summary. The inequality between states is the focus here, so the inequality between advantaged and disadvantaged kids is swept under the carpet by this model, statistically balanced as a fact of life that state administrators just have to accept. The statistical machinery behind this model isn't troubled by the apparent presumption that Black eighth graders are not as capable of mathematics, but in interpreting such a model, perhaps we should be. It's also a quirky counterfactual to contemplate—Vermont having the same racial mix as Alabama, or Hawaii having as many Spanish speakers as Texas. The math of this adjustment formula is nonchalant about such implications, of course, blithely inverting matrices without qualms, but it remains for us who wish to use the model to make sense of these assumptions—and to decide whether it really suits our purposes. And it is for us to live with its implications and messages, intended and otherwise.

Unfortunately, in these situations of considering adjusting or not adjusting a disparity, one must take a side. There is no neutral option. Consider a similar example about disparities in *child stunting*, a term describing children who are too short for their age because of nutritional deficiency. We often compare different countries by examining the frequency of stunting, which stands in as a measure of resources available to mothers and children and the success of antipoverty interventions.[18] This naturally leads to the question of how tall children *should be* at each age, and this standard is established by the World Health Organization (WHO) as an international consensus among well-nourished populations.[19] Using this standard, for example, nearly 40 percent of children in India are considered stunted.[20] But herein lies a dilemma because nutritional poverty is not the only determinant of child height. Rather, child height is highly correlated with maternal height, and Indian mothers are substantially shorter than those of other countries that make up the WHO standard. The average height of the mothers in other countries is 161.6 cm versus 151.7 cm for Indian mothers. Why are Indian mothers ten centimeters shorter? Of course it is because of nutritional deficiencies suffered when *they* were children, differences that are "baked in" to the current disparity, rather than a reflection of current nutritional policies affecting contemporary children.

Some researchers therefore standardize for maternal height to make a more "fair" comparison, effectively estimating what the stunting rate would be in India if, counter to fact, Indian mothers had the same height distribution as in other countries. When analyzed in this way, the prevalence of stunting in India is estimated as 25 percent rather than nearly 40 percent.[21] Similarly to the previous example with math exams, the disparities created by deprivation of mothers in the previous generation are excused by this adjustment, and instead, we get a more direct measure of how India is managing now, given the maternal height distribution that it has. This may be a fairer way of making a comparison with other countries, excusing past sins and focusing on the present, but it also misstates the factual proportion of kids who are too short—unless, of course, you view the short child of a short mother as beyond our control at the present time and, therefore, something better to be adjusted away, taken off the table. The point is that you can allow India the equivalent of a golf handicap if you most value fairness in the comparison with other countries, or you can insist on the absolute measure if you're instead after a realistic depiction of how tall Indian children are at any given age.

Here's another common sort of adjustment to think about: how to account for some people who are not actually at risk of an outcome. Over the past several decades, reported crime has been falling in the United States overall,[22] although the recent trends are less clear for violent crime. The COVID-19 pandemic and its associated restrictions on mobility seemed to have reduced violent crime in the United States in 2020 compared to 2019. But how does this relate to the risk of violent victimization experienced by individuals? Should I feel more safe or less safe venturing out of my house in 2020 than I did in 2019? The economists Maxim Massenkoff and Aaron Chalfin proposed that one should adjust for mobility in assessing change in risk.[23] The authors reasoned that if more people were staying locked up at home after March 2020, then the risk of victimization could be higher for those venturing out, even while overall incidence declined. So they adjusted the rate of violent crimes for the change in mobility of the population because they were interested in public violence and there were fewer people in public during lockdown. In crude numbers, public violence declined by 35 percent

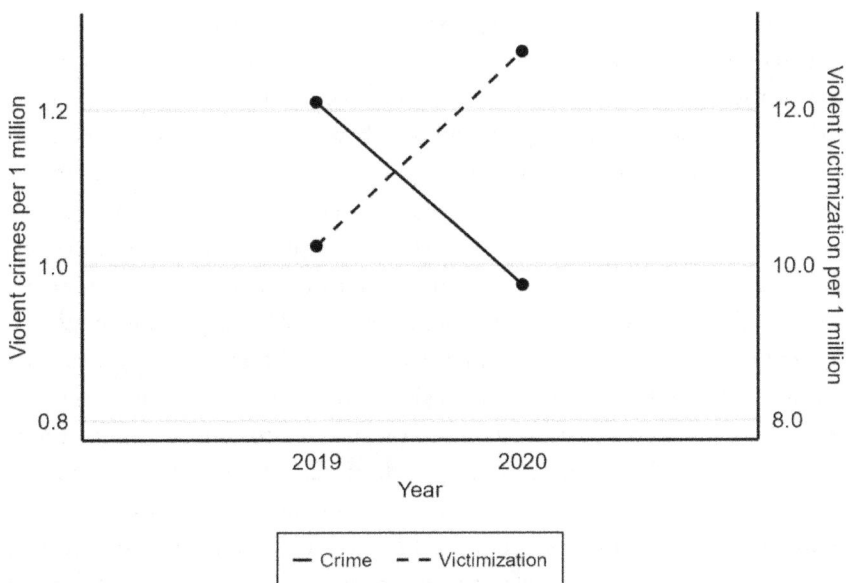

Figure 4.2 Trends in violent crime rates and violent victimization rates, 2019–2020

Source: Maxim Massenkoff and Aaron Chalfin, "Activity-Adjusted Crime Rates Show That Public Safety Worsened in 2020," *Proceedings of the National Academy of Sciences* 119, no. 46 (2022): e2208598119.

after March 2020, but time spent outside the home also decreased by 20 percent compared to 2019. The authors adjusted the number of violent crimes for time spent away from home so they could obtain the risk of street crime victimization for someone who ventures out. In their analysis, the adjusted risk of outdoor street crimes rose by more than 40 percent in the initial lockdown, ending up 24 percent higher by the end of 2020 (figure 4.2). It may seem something of a paradox that the number of violent incidents decreased while the risk to any individual in public increased, but one has to keep in mind that a rate is made of a numerator (number of events) and a denominator (people who are at risk to experience the event), and the pandemic affected both quantities. There is also something of a sleight of hand going on because the authors focus only on violence in public, ignoring the fact that people sheltering at home experienced greater risk of interpersonal violence from intimate partners and family members.[24]

The Massenkoff and Chalfin paper on violent victimization was not a paper about disparities between racial or ethnic groups, but a similar phenomenon occurs in that context too. This concern leads to a similar reliance on statistical adjustments for the population at risk: the denominator of the observed rate. Take the example of racial disparities in cervical cancer. Black women in the United States have a higher incidence of cervical cancer and worse survival once diagnosed.[25] In studies that estimate the risk of dying from cervical cancer, the measure used is the number of cervical cancer deaths divided by the number of people at risk of this outcome. People with male reproductive organs are not included in the denominator because they do not have a cervix and therefore cannot possibly appear in the numerator. The oncologist Anna Beavis and colleagues noticed that previously published surveillance of cervical cancer mortality inequalities had not taken into consideration the race-specific prevalence of hysterectomy, a surgical procedure that removes people with female anatomy from the population at risk of ever experiencing this outcome.[26] That is to say, a complete hysterectomy turns people with a cervix into people without a cervix, and this means that, after such a procedure, it becomes impossible to die of cervical cancer. Beavis and her colleagues therefore reasoned that because hysterectomy occurrence differs by race, these previous disparity studies had differentially mischaracterized the population at risk for the outcome and thus should be improved by statistical adjustment.

These authors obtained survey data on hysterectomy prevalence stratified by age, state, year, and race and used these values to reduce the sizes of the denominator populations to account for the proportions of Black and white women who were not actually at risk because of hysterectomies. Removing numbers from the denominator of a fraction makes the corrected values larger because deaths are divided by a smaller population at risk. The results reported by the authors were that for Black women, who have a higher prevalence of hysterectomy, the age-standardized mortality rate changed from 5.7 to 10.1 per 100,000 people per year. For white women, the age-standardized mortality rate changed from 3.2 to 4.7 per 100,000 people per year. The authors therefore noted that the previously uncorrected surveillance had underestimated the racial mortality disparity by more than 40 percent (figure 4.3).[27] They concluded that the previous literature has severely mischaracterized the magnitude of the racial injustice in cervical cancer mortality by differentially mischaracterizing the population that could actually experience the outcome. They also noted that the magnitude of this discrepancy increased with age because hysterectomy prevalence increases with age and rises more steeply in Black women than in white women.

White women

All ages:
Corrected = 4.7
Uncorrected = 3.2

·▲ Corrected ▬ Uncorrected

Annual mortality per 100,000 women

Age (years)

Black women

All ages:
Corrected = 10.01
Uncorrected = 5.7

·▲ Corrected ▬ Uncorrected

Annual mortality per 100,000 women

Age (years)

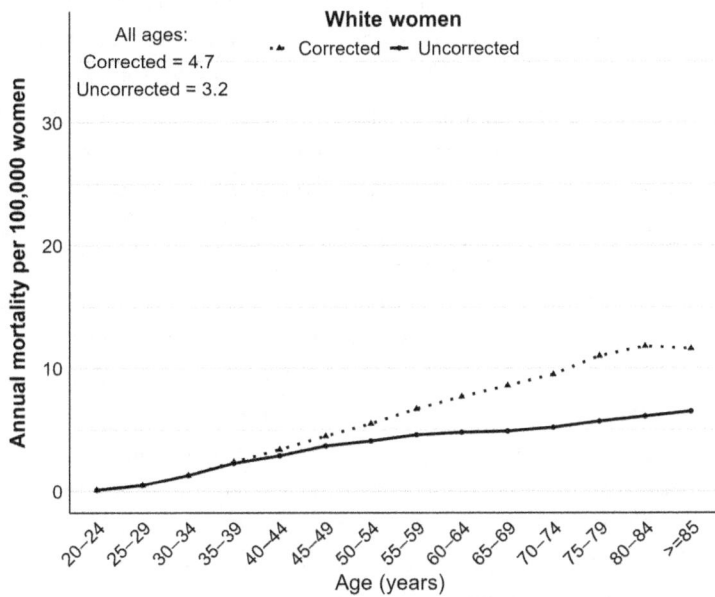

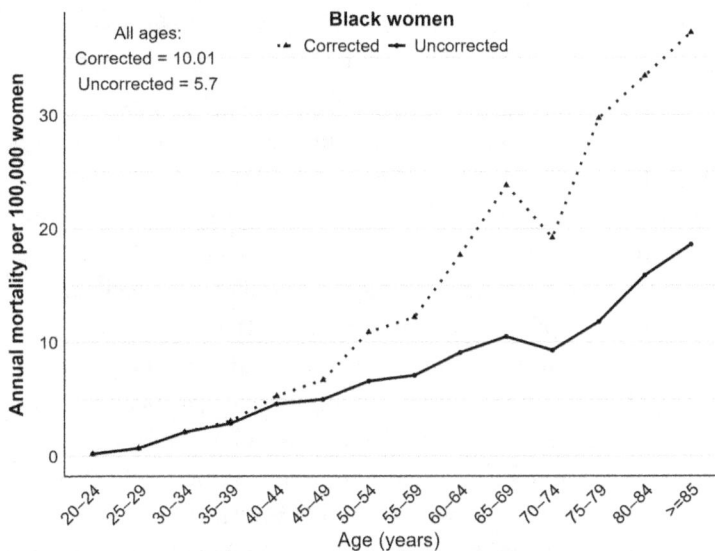

Figure 4.3 Annual U.S. cervical cancer mortality rates for Black and white women, by age, corrected or uncorrected for hysterectomy prevalence

Source: Anna L. Beavis, Patti E. Gravitt, and Anne F. Rositch, "Hysterectomy-Corrected Cervical Cancer Mortality Rates Reveal a Larger Racial Disparity in the United States," *Cancer* 123, no. 6 (2017): 1044–50.

The paper by Beavis and her colleagues is an astute work of descriptive epidemiology, and I see no significant technical flaws. It corrects an important deficiency in the previous literature and has been highly cited because of that. Nonetheless, the authors never discussed the ramifications of defining hysterectomy as a permissible covariate that should be adjusted and thus excused. The way it is treated in the paper, it seems like hysterectomy is just some mysterious fluke of nature that happens to strike some women and not others. But why should there be such a profound racial disparity in hysterectomy in the first place? And why should this be accepted nonchalantly as a given, rather than indicted as a further racial injustice? By making the statistical adjustment, the authors highlight how Black excess in cervical cancer deaths among those with a cervix had been understated. Paradoxically, a greater racial injustice is revealed by excusing away the underlying cause of that differential misclassification, which is the inexplicable excess of hysterectomies experienced by Black women. As analysts, we can't get away from the fact that adjustment may be warranted to bring one selected injustice into clearer focus at the same time that it removes some other injustice from view entirely. Statistical adjustment therefore functions as a kind of spotlight. When pointed at one problem, it can bring that problem more clearly into view. But adjacent issues are then cast into darkness, hidden from us.

There is another complication with the adjustment for hysterectomy, however, and this is that it ignores the fact that a complete hysterectomy really does prevent cervical cancer. Consider this horrific thought experiment. A surgeon performs a hysterectomy on all the Black women in a community, and thus the cervical cancer mortality rate among Black women in that population approaches zero because no Black women are at risk of the outcome. In this circumstance, the true racial disparity would be flipped: whites would have the higher rate of cervical cancer mortality. But would it still make sense to adjust for hysterectomy to pretend that they did not? The point is that the higher rate of hysterectomy in Black women is not a mere statistical artefact but a real component of the complete picture of racial disparity. People removed from the denominator are not "seen" by the resulting statistic, but they are still there in the real world, and adjustments of this kind necessarily obscure that fact. Or consider another way of looking at this issue, which is that there exists a vaccine against cervical cancer.[28] In reality, it is not 100 percent effective in eliminating incidence of the disease in the way that removing the cervix does, but it can come close if administered early in life. In a population with differential uptake of the vaccine by race, would we want to adjust away this difference and report the disparity only among those at risk because they had avoided vaccination? I suspect not because not being able to get the outcome is a real feature of the overall racial inequity in this outcome.

One can see this confusion even more overtly when looking at the press attention devoted to the Beavis article. The CNN headline was "Cervical Cancer Death Rates Are Much Higher Than Thought,"[29] which is clearly a false statement because the women with hysterectomies who were removed from the denominators of the rates were truly not getting cervical cancer. There was similar confusion at Newsmax, which proclaimed "Cervical Cancer Death Rates Shockingly Underestimated."[30] Again, the headline seems to take the adjusted rate as true and the crude rate as false, but in fact, it is the crude rate that actually exists in the real world. The adjusted rate might make for a fairer comparison between racial groups, although this too is up for debate. Beavis and colleagues thought it more relevant to report the death rates in a subset of women defined by hysterectomy status, which makes sense, but this is not what the news headlines state.

In this chapter, we have seen that adjustment procedures for racial and ethnic disparities rest on a different conceptual foundation from studies of treatment effects, even though they share the same mathematical procedures. The goal for observational studies of treatment effects is to mimic the randomized trial that we wish we could have conducted, the one in which all other variables are balanced between treatment arms.[31] For racial and ethnic disparities, however, there is no specific intervention in view, and the goal is instead a "fair" comparison of the group-specific measures. The crude (unadjusted) comparison reveals inequalities, simply whether one measure is larger or smaller than another. But these simple inequalities are rarely of interest because they can be accounted for by factors that we consider justifiable, such as different average ages. Having judged a cause of inequality to be acceptable, we can then remove it from view with a statistical adjustment, revealing the measures that would have been observed had this justifiable factor been balanced. In several real-world examples, we have seen that declaring ancillary factors to be permissible—and therefore candidates for adjustment—is not so simple. As analyses are conducted by different authors with different purposes or values, these adjustments will necessarily change. Moreover, removing a factor from view via adjustment can obscure inequities that are equally pernicious, even if they are not the focus of the analysis at hand. The adjustment can thus imply an acceptance of these excused factors as ethically inert, granting to them a sense of callous inevitability that the analysts may not really intend.

CHAPTER V

Conditional Disparities Are
the Devil's Playground

I n the two previous chapters, we paid a lot of attention to confounding, which is a bias due to a cause of the outcome that is correlated with but not affected by the treatment. In the context of studies documenting disparities between racial or ethnic groups, there may be no "treatment" in the literal sense, but we can still have a distortion akin to confounding if there are important covariates that are imbalanced between the groups being compared. This chapter considers another common source of statistical bias in the surveillance, prediction, and estimation of treatment effects, which is restriction or control for something affected by the treatment. In the context of studies examining racial and ethnic disparities, this would involve restriction or control for something affected by race and ethnicity. Because most social and material experiences are affected in some way by racial or ethnic identities, this bias can be a ubiquitous concern. This is somewhat more complicated to discuss than confounding because different academic disciplines describe this bias differently, have different names for it, or fail to recognize it at all. It generally receives less attention in most training programs and textbooks and yet can be a critically important problem for interpretation of causal and descriptive studies, including examination of racial and ethnic disparities. It is perhaps more conceptually subtle than confounding, and this is why it is more often overlooked in analytic corrections. More alarming is that many well-intentioned statistical corrections actually end up increasing this bias, and so this topic merits careful consideration.

Over the second half of the twentieth century, various statistical biases were recognized that involved the selection of participants into studies or the selective loss of some participants over time, and these were generally subsumed under a broad heading of *selection bias*.[1] These biases may best be understood as spurious associations that arise because of subsetting within a population. I refer to a *spurious association* as one that is distorted by some error, misattribution, or other anomaly. Subsetting occurs when one restricts attention to a selected subgroup through the study design (for example, recruiting only heart failure patients into the study) or when one restricts to some selected subgroup in the analysis (for example, fitting a statistical model among only those diagnosed with heart failure). It is this selecting in or out, whether by the analyst or the participants themselves, that gives rise to the term *selection bias*.[2]

The general understanding of these biases advanced considerably in the 1990s, with the new structural framework proposed by the computer scientist Judea Pearl. He developed graphical representations of causal relationships to demonstrate the consistent mechanisms of biases through configurations of nodes and arrows, as in the figures shown later in this chapter.[3] Pearl coined the term *collider variable* to refer to a quantity that has two causal inputs along some defined path, and he showed that conditioning in any way on such a variable can have surprisingly deleterious consequences. *Conditioning* is a broad statistical term: it can mean picking just one level of the variable or calculating the association measure at each level and then combining these together, which is essentially what a regression model does. Any conditioning on a collider variable, for example by conducting the analysis only among people diagnosed with a disease or adjusting for having the disease in a regression model, can lead to the problem that Pearl referred to as *collider stratification bias*. This was not widely appreciated until laid out so succinctly by Pearl in the 1990s. Miguel Hernán and colleagues proposed in 2004 that essentially all biases that epidemiologists had labeled as *selection biases* could be interpreted as collider stratification biases,[4] although this seems to have been an overstatement because some instances of selection bias have been described that clearly do not derive from collider stratification.[5]

In figure 5.1, consider a study on the relationship between COVID-19 vaccination and severe illness (left panel). Age is a confounder because it affects both treatment and outcome and so must be adjusted so that the estimated association is not distorted by confounding bias. Next, consider a study on the relation between age and COVID-19 vaccination (right panel).

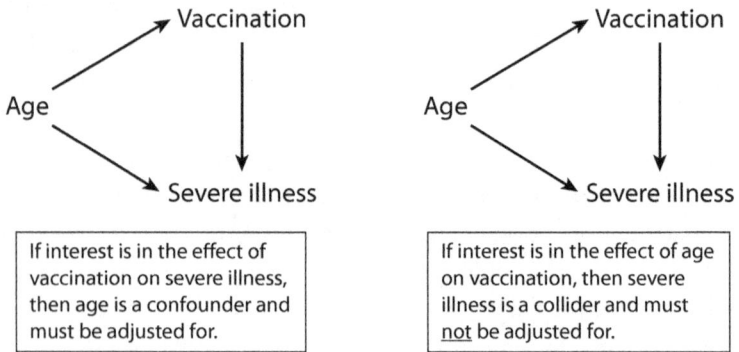

Vaccination   Vaccination

Age   Age

Severe illness   Severe illness

| If interest is in the effect of vaccination on severe illness, then age is a confounder and must be adjusted for. | If interest is in the effect of age on vaccination, then severe illness is a collider and must not be adjusted for. |

Figure 5.1 How the adjustment strategy depends on the scientific question: The example of age, vaccination status, and severe illness

These variables share the same relations with one another as in the left panel, but changing the scientific question also changes the analysis. Severe illness is affected by both the treatment and the outcome, and so it is a collider. It must not be adjusted for because doing so would incur collider stratification bias. This bias would occur, for example, if the study recruited disproportionately among those with severe illness or among those without severe illness.

To get an intuitive sense of what is going on with collider bias, consider the following example suggested by the epidemiologist Maria Glymour.[6] In the general population, there may be no particular correlation between height and athletic ability. If I know how tall someone is, it doesn't give me any information about how athletic they are. And if I know how athletic they are, I can't guess anything about their height. So these two quantities are unassociated within the general population, and therefore, one cannot predict or confound the other. But now zoom in to a highly selected subgroup like professional NBA players. There are two ways to get into this special club. You can either be very athletic, like Isaiah Thomas (5 feet, 9 inches tall), or you can just be outrageously tall, like Manute Bol (7 feet, 7 inches tall). Within this selected stratum of NBA players, therefore, the two traits are highly correlated and inversely so: taller NBA players tend to be less athletically talented, and shorter players tend to be more so (figure 5.2). The fact that these two variables are independent from one another in the real world but highly correlated in the NBA dataset is potentially catastrophic because it means that restrictions and adjustments can make analysis worse instead of better. Estimates could become worse, for instance, by distorting associations

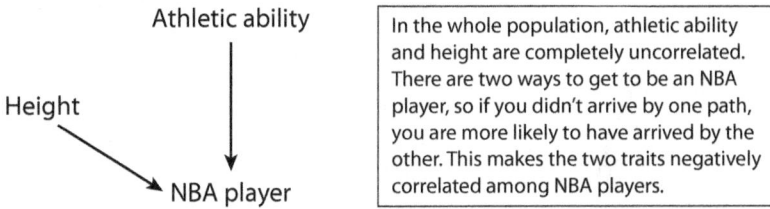

Athletic ability

Height

NBA player

> In the whole population, athletic ability and height are completely uncorrelated. There are two ways to get to be an NBA player, so if you didn't arrive by one path, you are more likely to have arrived by the other. This makes the two traits negatively correlated among NBA players.

Figure 5.2 How collider stratification produces a negative correlation between height and athletic ability among NBA players

between variables because correlated covariates cause confounding. Unfortunately, this kind of stratification happens in data collection, study design, and analysis all the time. This makes selection bias a constant potential danger, and yet awareness of this issue is only recently starting to catch up with the pervasiveness of the problem.[7]

How does this kind of collider stratification affect examination of racial and ethnic disparities? A striking example is the case of racial disparities in low birthweight. A healthy newborn at term should weigh between 2,500 and 4,000 grams, or between five and a half and nine pounds. We are concerned about newborns who weigh less than this because low birthweight is the leading risk factor for perinatal mortality. It has long been observed that Black Americans have lower birthweights than white Americans, with the whole distribution shifted down by around 200 grams.[8] But the curious observation, dating at least from the 1970s, is that the birthweight-specific risk curves plotted by race have a crossover (figure 5.3).[9] At normal birthweights, Black infants have a higher mortality risk, but among the smallest live births, those with weights below 2,500 grams, the risk of infant mortality is *lower* for Black infants.[10] A similar relationship is seen for mothers who smoke or don't smoke cigarettes during pregnancy, and this crossover in risk has been termed the *low birthweight paradox*.[11] What is paradoxical is simply that Black race puts infants at higher risk of mortality, and low birthweight puts infants at higher risk of mortality, but Black infants at low birthweights have *lower* risk of death than whites at the same birthweight. Several theories were floated over the years that this racial difference must be genetically determined and therefore that definitions of normal birthweight would have to be race specific to account for these hardwired differences.[12]

Although this paradox had nagged at researchers for decades, it took the recognition of the *collider bias* structure to finally solve the problem. In 2006,

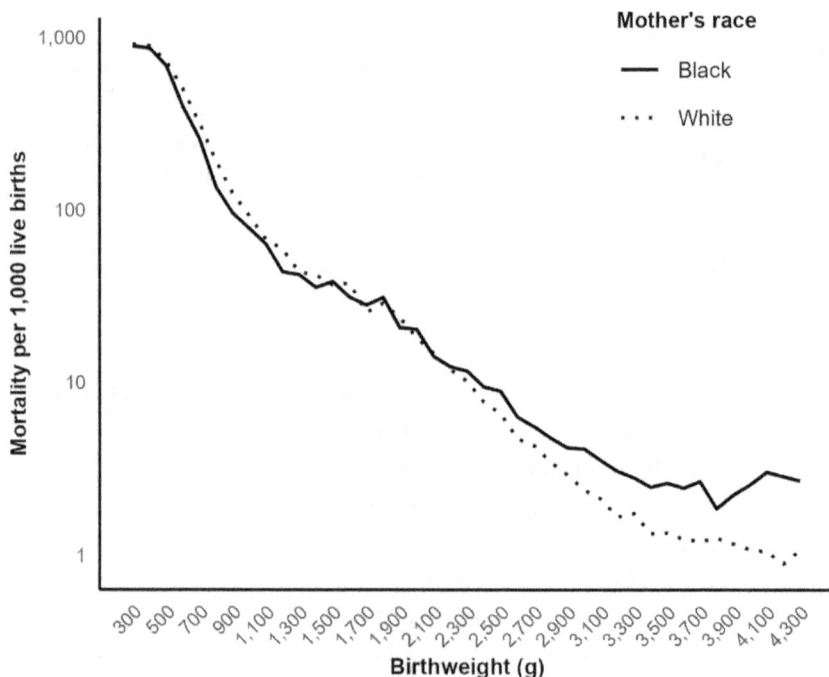

Figure 5.3 Infant deaths 2017–2021, showing the mortality crossover at 1,500–2,000 grams

Note: The vertical axis is on the log scale, so that the racial disparity in infant mortality is actually greater in magnitude at low birthweights than at high birthweights.

Source: Centers for Disease Control and Prevention, National Center for Health Statistics. National Vital Statistics System, Linked Birth/Infant Deaths on CDC WONDER Online Database. Data are from the Linked Birth/Infant Deaths Records 2017–2021, as compiled from data provided by the fifty-seven vital statistics jurisdictions through the Vital Statistics Cooperative Program. Accessed at http://wonder.cdc.gov/lbd-current-expanded .html on June 23, 2024, 6:50:56 PM.

epidemiologist Sonia Hernández-Díaz and colleagues unraveled the mystery by noting that the crossing mortality risk curves were conditional on birthweight, which was indeed a collider in this setting.[13] Remember that a Black infant with a low birthweight has a lower risk of death than a white infant *at the same birthweight*. It is this holding birthweight constant that is the conditioning behind the collider stratification bias.

To simplify the problem, think of just two pathways to low birthweight: Black race or a congenital anomaly (figure 5.4). These might be completely unrelated in the population so that no racial group is at any higher risk of a developmental fault that would slow fetal growth. If we observe that an

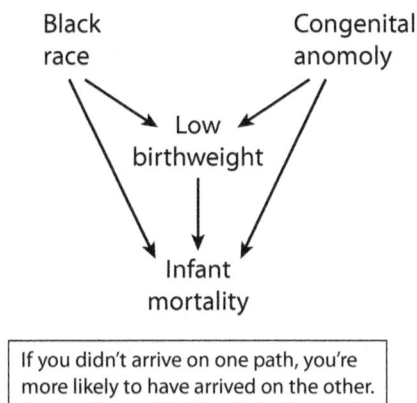

Figure 5.4 How collider stratification produces the low-birthweight paradox

infant is born with low birthweight, however, then the infant must have arrived at that outcome through one of the two pathways. If the infant is not Black, then they are more likely to have a congenital malformation that would explain the low birthweight. In this way, the two variables become confounded at each birthweight in a way that they are not confounded in the general population. This is problematic for the analysis because most causes of low birthweight and infant mortality are unknown and so the correlations induced by collider stratification cannot be easily adjusted away in any further analyses.[14]

The low birthweight paradox and its resolution make for a truly remarkable story because the mystery had been haunting the literature for decades, and all manner of complex physiological and evolutionary theories emerged to try to explain the observed patterns. When the solution finally came in 2006, it all turned out to be a very simple statistical error that was trivial to understand. It is hard to fathom that so much futile biological speculation swirled around a problem with such a simple statistical resolution, but hindsight is 20–20 as they say.[15] And it also doesn't mean that we're out of the woods just because we understand this structure. There is still no easy way to sort out adverse outcomes of pregnancy that arise from collider bias in more complex scenarios.

Take the example of racial disparity in the rate of neonatal death (which is the term for all deaths within four weeks of live birth). Babies are meant to gestate for around forty weeks, and coming out too early puts the newborn at higher risk. Because gestational age is such a powerful determinant of survival, we typically calculate neonatal death rates by week of gestational age, dividing the number of live-born children who die within twenty-eight days by the total number born at each week of gestation. Calculated in this way, the neonatal death rate for a Black preterm birth at twenty-eight to thirty-one weeks of gestation is 27.23 per 1,000 births, and for a white birth at this same gestational age, the rate is 32.73 per 1,000 births (table 5.1).[16] Despite Black babies having higher mortality overall and higher rates of preterm birth (which is the strongest mortality risk factor), the white death rate is 20 percent higher. Even understanding the collider structure shown earlier, it is not easy to make sense of how this disparity flips. But when we count the mortality rate not only in relation to all births at that gestational age but instead in relation to all infants still alive *whether already born or not at that moment*, then the preterm death rates become 0.35 and 0.19 per 1,000 ongoing pregnancies, or an 84 percent higher rate for Black preterm births.

The fact is that conditional disparities are just conceptually difficult. The way that racial disparity changes over the birthweight or gestational age distributions, when these factors are themselves affected by race, is not something that we have good intuitions about naturally, and there are many similar examples, including the so-called *obesity paradox*, which has a similar causal structure.[17] This is the observation that obesity is a risk factor for mortality, but among patients with a severe disease, like congestive heart failure, obesity appears to be protective. The lesson of these "paradoxes" is

TABLE 5.1

Counting neonatal mortality rates in relation to all births at each gestational age versus all infants still alive at each gestational age

Gestational age	Neonatal mortality rate per 1,000 preterm births			Neonatal mortality rate per 1,000 ongoing pregnancies		
	Black	White	Black/White	Black	White	Black/White
22–27 weeks	230.88	250.64	0.92	2.42	0.86	2.81
28–31 weeks	27.23	32.73	0.83	0.35	0.19	1.84
32–36 weeks	5.24	5.43	0.97	0.47	0.35	1.34

Source: Linked birth-infant death data files from the U.S. National Center for Health Statistics, 2014–2019, liveborn singletons, gestational age of 22–41 weeks without congenital anomalies.

to be very wary of racial or ethnic disparities examined within a stratum, where membership in that stratum is affected by race or ethnicity. That scenario is a misinterpretation disaster just waiting to happen, and that leads us naturally to our next example.

American police set a new record in 2022, killing 1,176 civilians, or roughly a hundred people per month.[18] Blacks make up 13 percent of the U.S. population but 24 percent of those killed by police in 2022, suggesting an important racial disparity in this outcome. Numerous papers in sociology, epidemiology, and economics have examined this phenomenon and its variation by location and evolution over time.[19] An important contribution to this evolving literature was a substantial research effort conducted by the economist Roland Fryer, published as a National Bureau of Economic Research report in 2016 and eventually as a peer-reviewed paper in a leading economics journal in 2019.[20] This extensive data collection and analysis involved a number of complementary datasets with large numbers of encounters with police and detailed covariate information on the police officers, the civilians, and the circumstances of their interaction. The published paper is more than fifty pages long and contains many findings across the various datasets. Some are perhaps not surprising, for example that Blacks and Hispanics were more than 50 percent more likely than whites to have an interaction with police that involved some use of force and that a racial disparity persisted even after controlling for more than a hundred covariates. But the result that was perhaps most unexpected and that garnered the most press attention was that in contrast to nonlethal uses of force, Fryer reported that, given an interaction with the police, there were no racial differences in officer-involved shootings.

The key qualifier for this finding is "given an interaction with the police." That is to say, the analysis conditions statistically on there being an encounter between the citizen and the police officer. This was necessary because the dataset was made up of encounters between citizens and the police, and so there was no accounting for the process of selecting people into those interactions. People obviously spend most of their lives not interacting with police officers, and so the data in the study are highly nonrepresentative of the overall population. Fryer addressed this concern head-on in his paper: "Understanding potential selection into police data sets due to bias in whom police interact with is a difficult endeavor," he explained. "Put simply, if one assumes that police simply stop whomever they want for no particular reason, there seem to be large racial differences. If one assumes they are trying to prevent violent crimes, then evidence for bias is small."[21] What does this mean? Fryer says that to interpret the relationship between a person's race and getting shot by the police once they are already having an encounter, one would have to consider how race might have gotten the person into that encounter in the first place.

Think of it this way. Suppose I am investigating potential racial disparities in skiing injuries in the United States. I go to a ski resort and collect demographic and injury data from those I find on the slopes, and I discover that the odds of experiencing an injury are higher for Black skiers than for white skiers. Can I go ahead and announce without further qualification that the Black population experiences a higher risk of skiing accidents? No, this would be entirely false because Blacks are substantially less likely to be skiing in the first place. Around 13 percent of the U.S. population identifies as Black, but a survey by the National Ski Areas Association found that this racial group made up less than 2 percent of skiers in 2020.[22] This means that, in fact, almost all skiing injuries will be among whites, even if we observe a higher rate among those Black people who are skiing.

Fryer had datasets of police encounters but no data on the characteristics of these people in relation to the general population from which they were selected and no information on what role, if any, race may have played in putting people into those encounters. If one assumes that race plays a role in that selection, then in fact there is evidence of racial bias in shootings in Fryer's data. But Fryer did not reach that conclusion because he was not willing to assume that police are racist in giving any selective attention to minorities. Rather, he assumed that police respond to requests for assistance and to legitimate indications of criminality and therefore engage with civilians in a way that is free from racial prejudice. On the basis of this benefit of the doubt, Fryer concluded that he found "no evidence of racial discrimination in officer-involved shootings."[23] In sum, it is only by assuming as a premise that police are free from racial bias in selecting to encounter someone that Fryer could conclude that police are free from racial bias in their decision to shoot that person.

The structure of this problem is very similar to the other selection bias examples described earlier, like the low birthweight paradox. Recall that among babies born underweight, the causes of arriving at that condition were negatively correlated, so that if a baby didn't arrive via one mechanistic pathway, they were more likely to arrive by another. A similar thing happens in the selected subset of police interactions. Suppose there are two ways to

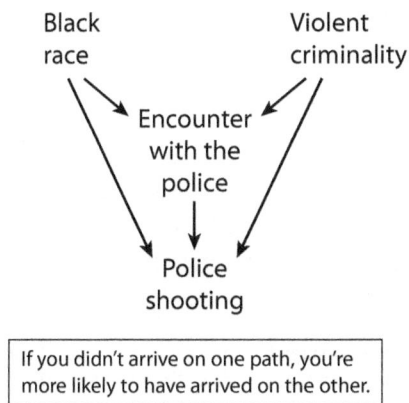

```
        Black                    Violent
        race                   criminality
            \                   /
             \                 /
              ↘  Encounter  ↙
                 with the
                  police
                    ↓
                 Police
                 shooting
```

```
┌─────────────────────────────────────────┐
│ If you didn't arrive on one path, you're  │
│ more likely to have arrived on the other. │
└─────────────────────────────────────────┘
```

Figure 5.5 How collider stratification produces a spuriously lower risk of police shooting among Black citizens

get stopped by the police, either by being Black or by exhibiting the behavior of a criminal (figure 5.5). Even if these are completely uncorrelated in the wider world, they will be negatively correlated among those detained by the police, so that violent criminals will be disproportionately non-Black and Blacks will be disproportionately noncriminal, relative to their representations in the general population. In such a setting, it would therefore not be surprising to observe that Black race is *protective against police shooting*, but this would not signal an absence of racial bias among police. Rather, it would simply result from the population of detained individuals being watered down by many noncriminals who are stopped excessively exactly because of the racial bias of the police. In this setting, therefore, the rate of police shootings of Blacks can be elevated at the population level due to racial bias, even while appearing to be lower in this analysis due to conditioning on the encounter and assuming that this is not due to racial bias, as Fryer has done.

If you step through the diagram with numbers, you can see more concretely how the apparently protective effect of Black race arises from conditioning on encounters with the police. Start with a fictitious population of 1,000 people, 20 percent of whom are Black and 5 percent of whom are violent criminals (figure 5.6). Race and criminality are completely uncorrelated in our example, so the proportion of Black criminals would be just the simple product of $0.20 \times 0.05 = 0.01$, and thus 1 percent of the total population are Black criminals, equal to $0.01 \times 1,000 = 10$ individuals. Now suppose that the police are very good at their job, and so they encounter

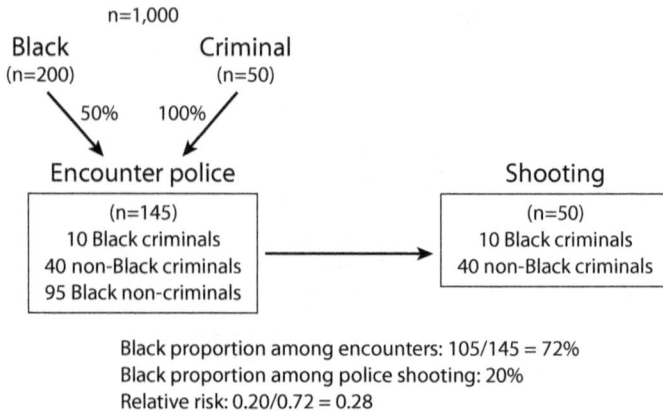

```
                          n=1,000
            Black                    Criminal
           (n=200)                    (n=50)
                 50%        100%
                    ↘      ↙
            Encounter police                        Shooting
        ┌─────────────────────┐              ┌─────────────────────┐
        │      (n=145)        │              │      (n=50)         │
        │  10 Black criminals │   ────────▶  │  10 Black criminals │
        │ 40 non-Black criminals│            │ 40 non-Black criminals│
        │ 95 Black non-criminals│            └─────────────────────┘
        └─────────────────────┘
```

Black proportion among encounters: 105/145 = 72%
Black proportion among police shooting: 20%
Relative risk: 0.20/0.72 = 0.28

Figure 5.6 A numerical demonstration of how restricting to police encounters produces a spuriously lower risk of police shooting among black citizens

100 percent of the criminals. But they are also very racist in their suspicions, and so they also encounter 50 percent of the Black population. In that case, the population of police encounters is 145, made up of 50 criminals (10 Black and 40 non-Black) plus 95 Black noncriminals. Now let's also give the police the benefit of the doubt and assume that they only ever shoot criminals. The total number shot is therefore 50, of which 10 are Black.

From this simple scenario, we can observe that the Black proportion among the police encounters is 105/145 = 72 percent and the Black proportion among the shootings is 20 percent, which is exactly their share of the total population. There is no racial bias in police shooting in this example, but if you make the error of conditioning on police encounters, then the risk appears to be only 10/145 = 7 percent. The relative risk for Blacks to be involved in police shootings is therefore 0.20/0.72 = 0.28, making Black race look highly protective, even though it is not.

It is perhaps not surprising that the media devoted great attention to this unexpected finding. "How a Controversial Study Found That Police Are More Likely to Shoot Whites, Not Blacks" read a headline in the *Washington Post*.[24] The conservative media was even more delighted, with the *Washington Times* headline declaring "No Racial Bias in Police Shootings, Study by Harvard Professor Shows."[25] It is also unsurprising that none of this coverage noted the conditional disparity because this is a statistical subtlety that is easily overlooked by most journalists and newspaper readers. Some responsibility for this confusion must also be shared by Fryer, who was meticulous in the academic paper about stressing the conditional disparity as a caveat but does not explain this issue or make the same caveats in his media interviews. In fact, Fryer told the *New York Times* that the protective effect of Black race against police shooting was "the most surprising result of [his] career,"[26] which seems a strange sentiment for someone who clearly understood the statistical implications of studying the conditional disparity while explicitly assuming no racial bias in police interaction with Black citizens.

Conditioning on having an encounter with the police is a form of adjustment, just like the statistical adjustments that we have discussed in previous chapters. In effect, Fryer's paper adjusts away the effect of excess police interaction with Black citizens, looking only at the disparity in shooting that arises *given* such excess interaction, rather than the disparity in shooting that might arise *because* of this excess interaction. I don't find any clear discussion in the paper about a justification for this adjustment, but Fryer seems to imply that it would be unfair to compare crude shooting rates between race groups because Blacks and Hispanics simply have more opportunity to be shot due to their much more frequent encounters with police. Even so, I believe strongly that adjusting this difference away is misleading in relation to what people really want to understand about the disparity. The conditional contrast simply doesn't answer the real motivating question. For example, suppose my doctor tells me that I am too sedentary and so I need to join a gym and exercise more. Later he asks me if I have followed this recommendation. It would be clearly disingenuous of me to provide a conditional response: "Whenever I am at the gym, I spend more time exercising than being sedentary." It may be a true statement, but it doesn't really answer the question, and my doctor wouldn't be fooled.

Neither was the academic community fooled by the analysis of police shootings. A number of critics in sociology, political science, and economics quickly pounced on the Fryer paper, issuing critiques of the methodology and interpretation. Notable among these were a series of papers by the political scientists Dean Knox and Jonathan Mummolo in which they carefully examined the conditional methodology and showed that it simply could not answer relevant questions about racial bias in policing.[27] These critiques were largely ignored by Fryer, but similar concerns were expressed in 2020 by the economists Steve Durlauf and James Heckman, which finally provoked a response.[28] Fryer published a rebuttal in which he insisted that he had made no claims whatsoever about racial discrimination or racial bias in his paper and only documented "racial differences" and, furthermore, that he had duly warned readers about the conditional analysis and the assumption of no racial bias in selecting civilians into police encounters.[29] These caveats and disclaimers are indeed readily evident in the published academic work, but they are completely absent from the media discussions, including in interviews with Fryer himself.[30] The 2019 paper by Fryer is still embraced uncritically as evidence that Black and Hispanic men are not at higher risk of police shootings than white men, such as in a recent review of this question published by the right-wing Manhattan Institute.[31]

One should also keep in mind that the 2019 Fryer paper, although it received a lot of media and academic attention, was not the only study to make this common error. For example, a 2019 paper by the psychologist David Johnson and his colleagues in the *Proceedings of the National Academy of Sciences* used a dataset of police shootings in which they had information on officer and civilian race and similarly claimed that there were no excess police shootings of Black and Hispanic citizens by white officers.[32] After pointed criticism by Knox and Mummolo,[33] the authors took the uncommonly principled step to retract their paper,[34] stating, "A critique pointed out we had erroneously made statements about racial differences in the probability of being shot, and we issued a correction to rectify the statement. Despite this correction, our work has continued to be cited as providing support for the idea that there are no racial biases in fatal shootings, or policing in general. To be clear, our work does not speak to these issues and should not be used to support such statements."[35]

The retraction of the Johnson et al. paper, however, raises troubling questions about political guardrails placed on statistical malfeasance. After all, most data sources across all of the social and biomedical sciences involve selected cohorts. The worst instances are large projects like the UK Biobank, in which about 95 percent of invitations were refused, making the study sample dramatically richer, older, leaner, healthier, and female than the British population from which it arose.[36] The UK Biobank is also notable because, as of the end of 2022, it had already given rise to more than six thousand published scientific papers.[37] Must all of these papers be tossed out? In fact, retraction of published scientific papers remains exceedingly rare and usually occurs not because the analysis was faulty but only because overt fraud is detected. A right-wing think-tanker named Heather Mac Donald, the author of a 2016 book *The War on Cops*, leveled the accusation that the paper by Johnson and colleagues was retracted because she had used it as evidence in a congressional hearing and in newspaper editorials defending the conduct and integrity of police officers.[38] In fact, the retraction was requested by the authors themselves, and they insisted that retraction was necessitated by their own erroneous interpretation in the published paper. But they also mentioned the need for retraction because of how it was used in public debates by those generally on the political right who wished to exonerate the police. The journal took the unusual additional step of including an editorial that accompanied the retraction, in which the editors described why the selection bias problem invalidates the stated interpretation.[39] Nonetheless, like Fryer, they proposed that perhaps the findings might be a valid description of racial differences in the victim pool, even if these numbers are not relevant to the broader question of racial bias in police shooting that the authors claimed to be addressing. Rather than allow for this admittedly more convoluted interpretation, the editors wrote that the paper should be retracted specifically because of the misuse of the article, including its citation by Heather Mac Donald in a *Wall Street Journal* article titled "The Myth of Systemic Police Racism."[40] What can we conclude from this whole incident? At the very least, it seems necessary to concede that all errors are not equal. Some do more social harm than others.

Selection bias occurs in countless similar situations when observations are selected *into* the dataset, like in the example of shootings that occur during interactions with the police. These situations are so routine that once you recognize the general pattern, it is hard not to see it almost everywhere. I challenged myself to flip through the articles in a recent issue of the *Journal of the American Medical Association* (*JAMA*), and sure enough, I stumbled across a perfect example of this phenomenon almost immediately. The health policy scholar Marian Jarlenski and colleagues extracted data on drug testing among almost 38,000 pregnant women during labor and delivery in a large healthcare system in Pennsylvania.[41] They reported on receipt of the test and result of the test by mother's race, adjusting for covariates including age, ethnicity, and tobacco use. White women had a much higher proportion of positive drug screens. Among those with a self-reported history of substance abuse, for example, 66.7 percent of white women tested positive compared to 58.3 percent of Black women. Does this mean that white women had more drug use during pregnancy? No, and the reason it doesn't is that we have data only on the women selected into testing. If testing was random, then we would know the prevalence of drug use in the population of pregnant women, but in fact, it turned out to be far from random, with a racial disparity that was not explained by the legitimate indications for testing. Among those women without a substance abuse history, 6.9 percent of Black women were tested compared to 4.7 percent of white women. Likewise, among those with a substance abuse history, which is considered a legitimate indication to warrant a test, 86.4 percent of Black women were tested compared to 68.7 percent of white women (figure 5.7). Therefore, Black women were differentially surveilled for "bad" behaviors during pregnancy, just as Black citizens were differentially brought into police encounters in the previous example. As a result, we can expect a racial disparity in the testing results, even if there is no racial disparity in drug use in the population.

The examples above, such as encounters with police and drug testing of pregnant women, involve differential selection *into* the dataset. But bias also occurs in many situations by selectively dropping observations *out* of the dataset, as in the case of people exiting from the follow-up period in longitudinal studies for reasons related to the treatment. One common reason that people drop out of long follow-ups is because they die, which is a problem referred to as one of *competing events*.[42] For example, consider that smoking prevents Alzheimer's disease, a disease of the central nervous system that leads to memory loss and dementia.[43] Risk of Alzheimer's disease increases markedly with advanced age, and smoking selects people out of advanced aging by having them die earlier from lung cancer and cardiovascular disease. Although we want to avoid ever getting Alzheimer's disease, dying of something else first is generally not the way we want to avoid it. This suggests that when we study this relationship, what most people really want to know is something more complicated, like how smoking would hypothetically impact Alzheimer's disease if we could somehow prevent people from dying from the diseases of smoking.[44]

Similarly confusing scenarios arise when we consider racial and ethnic differences in overall mortality by age because the populations become increasingly selected by mortality as age advances. This leads to a paradoxical crossing of mortality curves for racial groups, not unlike the crossing mortality curves we saw in the low birthweight example.[45] For example, overall rates of mortality are higher for Blacks than for whites in the United States, but if you consider the contrast of mortality rates at each age, there is a flip around eighty years of age, after which Blacks have the *lower* mortality rate (figure 5.8). This is consistently observed, and there are

A. Urine toxicology test

B. Positive toxicology test result

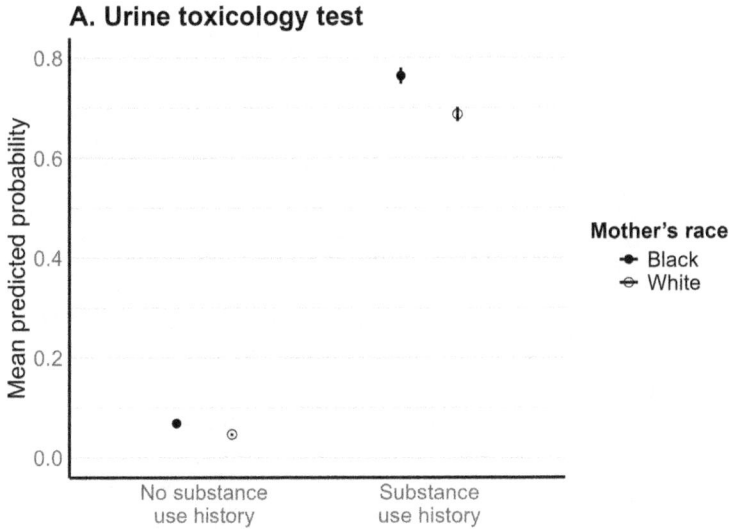

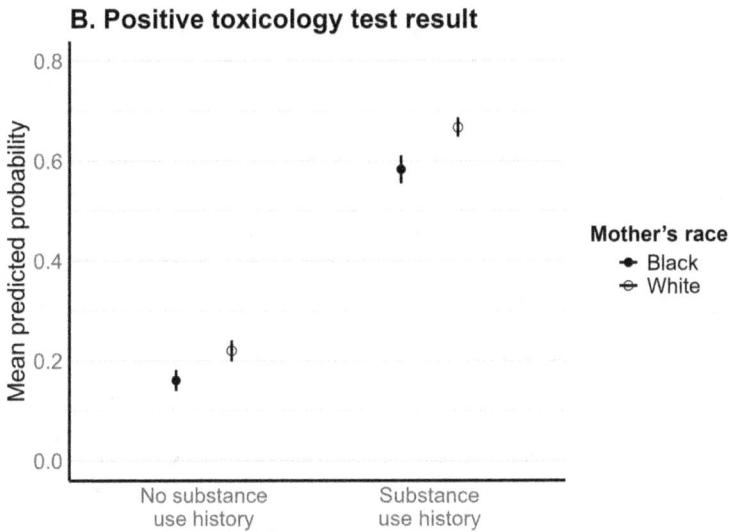

Figure 5.7 Association of race with urine toxicology testing and results among pregnant patients during labor and delivery

Source: Marian Jarlenski et al., "Association of Race with Urine Toxicology Testing Among Pregnant Patients During Labor and Delivery," *JAMA Health Forum* 4 (2023): e230441, https://www.doi.org/10.1001/jamahealthforum.2023.0441.

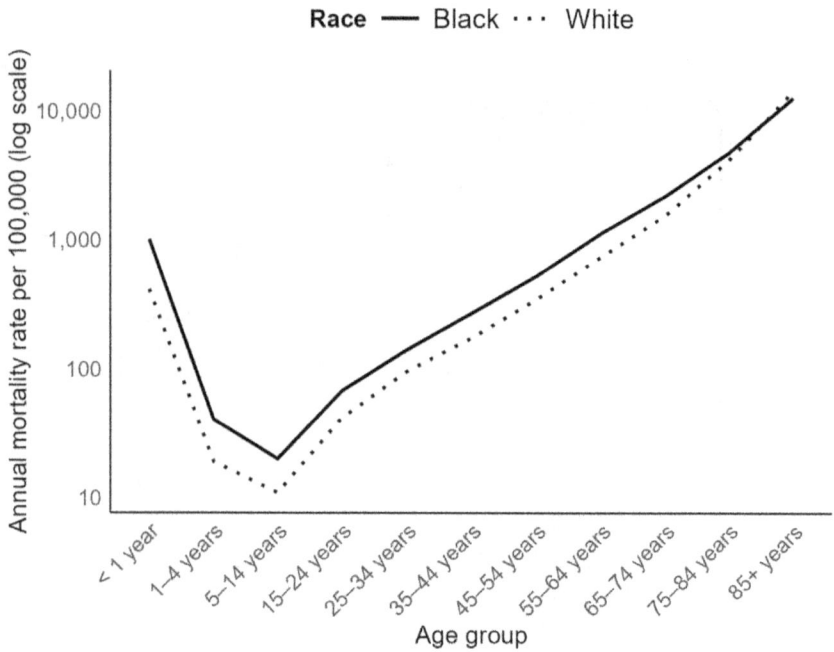

Figure 5.8 Mortality rates by age groups and race, women, United States, 2018–2022

a number of ways to make sense of this phenomenon. It can be viewed as just another instance of collider stratification bias, where the collider is survival to each specific age, and we condition on that collider by comparing age-specific mortality rates. Equivalently, this phenomenon can be seen as a kind of continual depletion of the most fragile portion of the population, such that the remaining population becomes enriched with only the most resilient members.

It is very easy to demonstrate this phenomenon numerically, adapting a simple example provided by the physician Steve Stovitz and colleagues.[46] Take a cohort of one hundred people with three categories of genetically determined longevity, such that 20 percent have a short life expectancy of sixty years, 60 percent have a medium life expectancy of eighty years, and 20 percent have a long life expectancy of one hundred years. Moreover, there is a racial disparity in life expectancy, such that Black individuals, who make up 30 percent of the cohort, have a life expectancy ten years shorter than white participants, due to systemic racism, even though the proportions of longevity genes are equal in the two race groups. From these proportions

TABLE 5.2

A fictitious example of expected lifespans among a cohort of one hundred people with three levels of genetic predisposition and a racial disparity

| | Genetic potential | | | |
	Short life	Medium life	Long life	
Black	50 (n = 6)	70 (n = 18)	90 (n = 6)	n = 30
White	60 (n = 14)	80 (n = 42)	100 (n = 14)	n = 70
	n = 20	n = 60	n = 20	n = 100

above, we can deduce the expected lifespans of the one hundred individuals, as shown in table 5.2.

Therefore average lifespan among the Black participants will be:

$$[(6 \times 50) + (18 \times 70) + (6 \times 90)]/30 = 2{,}100/30 = 70 \text{ years.}$$

And average lifespan among the white participants will be:

$$[(14 \times 60) + (42 \times 80) + (14 \times 100)]/70 = 5{,}600/70 = 80 \text{ years.}$$

So far so good, and the ten-year life expectancy deficit for Black participants is evident in the average lifespans. But now comes the surprising crossover. Monitor the racial disparity as the cohort ages. What does it look like after age seventy? By that point, we have lost those with lifespans of fifty, sixty, and seventy years, which is to say, all of those with the short longevity genes and the Black participants with medium longevity genes. At this point, in the remaining population, we observe:

The average lifespan among the six remaining Black participants =
$$(6 \times 90)/6 = 90 \text{ years.}$$

And average lifespan among the fifty-six remaining white participants =
$$[(42 \times 80) + (14 \times 100)]/56 = 4{,}760/56 = 85 \text{ years.}$$

There is a crossover because in the remaining cohort, the Black participants now live longer than the white participants. In fact, no individual Black person ever lives longer because they are Black because the effect of systemic racism removes ten years of life expectancy from all Black participants uniformly. But conditional on remaining in the cohort past age seventy, Blacks will have better genes than whites, even though the genetic potential was equal at the start of the cohort. This can also be viewed as collider stratification, in which race and genes are the two causes of exiting the cohort. These two factors were uncorrelated at the beginning of follow-up but become highly correlated by age seventy due to the selective attrition. Indeed, this is an inevitable characteristic of all follow-up studies: even if they are randomized so that covariates are perfectly balanced at the start of the follow-up, they will become increasingly unbalanced as people start to leave the cohort either because they die or are lost to follow-up. This means that a randomized trial does not stay randomized for very long.[47]

In sum, conditional disparities are a persistently confusing topic, and a more detailed examination of this problem requires a level of statistics beyond what can be conveyed in this book. What is most important to look for in evaluating studies critically is the restriction to a subgroup whose membership is somehow affected by the factors of interest. For instance, when considering the causal effect of smoking on Alzheimer's disease in a cohort of aging participants, are people dropping out of the study differentially by smoking? Likewise, for racial and ethnic disparities, the problem comes if people are selected into or out of the study based on race or ethnicity, for example by being selected into encounters with the police, or out of follow-up by differential mortality rates. This is a red flag that selection bias might distort the results. Similarly, be wary of "convenience samples" that might involve considerable self-selection into participating, as one might find in online surveys or studies of volunteers.[48] There are analytic techniques for trying to overcome these selection problems, but they require some stronger assumptions and more elaborate modeling and are still all too rare among published scientific papers in all disciplines.

CHAPTER VI

The Mismeasure of Man

T‍he title of this chapter invokes the famous 1981 book by the pale-ontologist Stephen J. Gould, in which he critiqued the statistical methods that were used to demonstrate racial differences in traits like intelligence.[1] Gould's book spurred my initial interest in the topic of racial differences when it was assigned to me as a supplementary reading in an introductory biostatistics class in the 1980s, although the text is primarily focused on psychology and psychometrics. Nonetheless, the issue of measurement is central to Gould's book because intelligence cannot be directly observed and so must instead be estimated, usually from various test questions, the results of which are then combined through the alchemy of statistics into a single measure that supposedly represents general intelligence. The very existence of such a trait is itself controversial, but even allowing that it may exist, estimating it from test items necessitates additional layers of uncertainty and debate.[2] The science of concrete things, like geology and chemistry, is challenging enough. Things get much trickier when the object under study isn't an object at all but an abstraction, one that can be glimpsed only obliquely with measures cobbled together from indicators whose relationship to the target is imperfect, perhaps substantially so.

Classification and measurement errors of one form or another are ubiquitous across all branches of science, but how these are dealt with varies widely by discipline. Educational research, for example, tends to expend great effort to model measurement errors for assessments of student performance, whereas similar corrections in economics are relatively rare. But these fields also exemplify completely different kinds of target quantities: the psychological constructs are almost completely abstract and thus ultimately unverifiable. You can't cut someone open to see how much neuroticism or cynical hostility they really have inside them. The best you can do is find measures that are reliable, in the sense of generating similar estimates from one examination to the next. These test items ought to also have some kind of "face validity" in that they seem to match the trait being targeted. In economics, by contrast, the quantities of interest tend to be concrete and verifiable things like wages and expenditures. There are still potential errors in the recorded values because people may misreport or miscalculate, but validation is at least feasible in principle.

Epidemiology probably falls somewhere between these extremes. Many exposures are concrete entities like chemicals or viruses, but measurement of behaviors like smoking and physical activity can fail to capture a wide range of variations that lead to very different effective dosages of the etiologically relevant experiences. There are also huge differences in the impact of measurement error depending on the exposure. Nutritional research is among the most challenging. Habitual diet is clearly relevant to chronic disease outcomes like cancer and heart disease, and so this branch of epidemiology is a major part of essential public health science. And yet measures of habitual diet generally come from surveys in which people report how much of everything they ate in, say, the last twenty-four hours. It's no surprise that people are not very good at this kind of task, nor is what a person ate in the last twenty-four hours a particularly good measure of one's overall diet.[3] The same applies to studies of exercise, drinking, and other health behaviors for which self-report is often far from the mark and sometimes correlated with other factors (for example, heavier people tend to underestimate their habitual caloric intakes and lighter people tend to overestimate).[4]

Epidemiological outcomes are prone to being more abstract because what constitutes a "disease" is often an arbitrary cut point along some continuous function. For example, the medical condition labeled as "hypertension" is a chronic elevation of blood pressure and a leading cause of stroke and cardiovascular disease. But blood pressure fluctuates constantly, and hypertension is defined based on a completely arbitrary threshold, like 140 millimeters of mercury displaced. One is not perfectly healthy at 139 mmHg and suddenly gravely ill at 141 mmHg. But medicine needs cut-off points to trigger diagnoses and treatments, and so where nature provides a continuum, humans impose an imaginary bright line. Other diseases can be even more abstract, not only because of the cut-off problem but because the function under study is more complex, multidimensional, or vague. For instance, how can we know who really has depression or attention deficit disorder or autism? How many people are incorrectly diagnosed with these kinds of conditions? How many are incorrectly *un*diagnosed? In many such cases, without a concrete standard, we cannot create effective validation studies that might inform the necessary statistical adjustments and corrections.

A great number of statistical approaches do exist for addressing classification errors, but these generally require some consensus about the true value, against which the recorded measure can be checked and compared. For example, when we diagnose some people to have a disease and others to be free of disease, we risk two kinds of errors. The first is labeling truly sick people as free of disease, and the second is mistaking truly well people as having the disease. In clinical medicine, these errors are governed by the *sensitivity* and *specificity* of the diagnostic test. Sensitivity is defined as the proportion of truly diseased people who are correctly labeled by the test as diseased, and specificity is the proportion of those truly free of disease who are correctly classified as not having the disease. A diagnostic test that is 100 percent sensitive and 100 percent specific will make neither error, but such tests are rare if they exist at all. For example, the Pap smear,[5] which is the common screening test for cervical cancer, has a sensitivity of roughly 55 percent and a specificity of about 97 percent. That means that if you really don't have cervical cancer, this test will falsely claim that you do about 3 percent of the time. But if you truly do have cervical cancer, the test will claim that you don't almost half the time.[6] Clinical researchers conduct validation studies to determine the sensitivity and specificity of various diagnostic tests, but these all presume the existence of a gold standard as a basis to define the truth. When a variable is abstract rather than concrete, perhaps something that is not even real, then no gold standard can possibly exist, and quantifying the measurement error becomes much more complicated and potentially controversial.

Unfortunately, this is where things stand in relation to racial and ethnic disparities because these imagined subclassifications of human beings are also vague and their boundaries are set by arbitrary administrative definitions that shift over time and place. Human traits—from height to skin color—tend to vary along continua. The construction of human subgroups in which people have one identity versus another across some bright line is a social convention, not a feature of the natural world. The difficulties associated with assignment of people into these boxes are frequently ignored in applied work and in the routine reporting by government and institutions, presumably because there is no objective solution, given that the divisions are not natural entities subject to verification. One could imagine making less ambiguous groupings according to one naturally categorical physical trait. For example, one could decide to define "races" of human beings according to their ABO blood groups, and then we would have a more concrete and verifiable classification system. But, unfortunately for us, this is not the kind of classification system we have. Instead, our racial and ethnic designations are historically and politically determined markers of identity and affiliation. Because identity cannot be directly observed by others, the only way to ascertain a person's identity is to ask them.[7] This means that the answers people provide can legitimately change over time for the same individual as they discover a new identity or over time within families as they evolve new social positions.[8] It also means that if someone claims an identity, there is no way to prove the claim is true or false.

The absence of a gold standard for race means that there can be no confirmatory blood test or genetic marker, and classifications can be highly variable from person to person, from place to place, and from time to time. This arbitrariness can be witnessed in the chaotic checkboxes of the U.S. decennial census, which in 1890 counted Mulattos, Quadroons, and Octoroons, but by 1980 considered all of these people to be simply "Black," and instead separated out Hawaiians, Samoans, and Guamanians as distinct responses.[9] Classifications of identity and affiliation are inherently fluid, and although they may be correlated with ancestry and physical appearance in some familiar ways, the best we can do is to try to predict how people might classify themselves. In principle, we can never assert that any self-definition is false because there are no objective boundaries on group membership. In practice, there are constraints of social perception that place limits on which identity claims will be embraced by others, with people at the margins of physical trait distributions having the most latitude.[10]

Governments that monitor racial and ethnic disparities must set down administrative definitions of groups, but there is no guarantee that these official definitions will match the self-identity of any individual. For example, there are now roughly five million Americans who trace their ancestry to the Indian subcontinent. These people are classified by the federal government as "Asian American," yet when researchers polled this population and asked whether they consider themselves Asian American, fewer than half did. Likewise, Arab Americans were classified as "white" in the census and for all administrative purposes such as monitoring diversity until 2024, even though, when polled, less than a third of this group identified as white.[11] This recent splitting off of "Middle East and North Africa," or MENA, identities from the broader white group illustrates how boundaries between groups inevitably shift over time in relation to political lobbying, characteristics of immigrants, and political events. The impetus for the new MENA category arose in part from the fallout of the 9/11 attacks in 2001 and the subsequent war in Iraq, leading to Arab Americans generally feeling less welcome as "white" than they had before.[12]

Biomedicine has long been uncomfortable with self-reported racial categorizations exactly because they are potentially subjective and unstable. Therefore, it has been increasingly proposed in the clinical literature that these be substituted with genetic ancestry estimated from DNA.[13] This is now a commonly applied technology in cohort and biobank studies in which genotyping is available. By using a large number of variants across the genome, the test can characterize the donor in relation to frequencies of these traits in reference populations. This procedure allows us to classify a person in terms of continuous degrees of membership in any number of latent categories representing hypothetical ancestries, defined in relation to contemporary samples taken from around the globe. Note that these target groupings are inherently *latent*, which means that they can be estimated but never directly observed. The exact number and even the very existence of such categories are merely conjectures. The statistical procedure provides estimated probabilities of membership in these imagined groups, without in any way implying that the divisions are real. If the analyst asks for more groups or fewer groups, the results will differ, and yet there is no objective justification to hypothesize any specific number of such groups. It's like asking how many distinct colors there are in the rainbow. Because the wavelength of radiation can take any value, there is in principle an infinite number of colors, and humans may be capable of distinguishing more than a million distinct shades. In practice, however, we group these much more crudely. No grouping is inherently more true than another.

Thanks to sexual reproduction, humans are a bit lumpier than light waves, however, and so there are people more closely and distantly related to each other. This lets us consider how much variation there is in any trait or collection of traits within some group compared to how much there is between these groups. But one can detect this kind of structure at every level of aggregation. Asked to divide humanity into four to six groups, genetic clustering algorithms tend to segregate roughly by continents because oceans have presented at least some challenge to gene propagation.[14] Because people tend to be more similar to those nearby, looking within continental populations also reveals finer structure, and here we can see how people have segregated themselves into national and regional patterns of endogamy.[15] Zooming in further to any national or ethnic population with enough geographic or social variation, one finds structure here too, as people prefer their romance to be relatively more local and familiar.[16] Ancestry is therefore as much of a continuum as any other human characteristic, and the categories we use are therefore to some extent always necessarily arbitrary. As time passes, some identities become more or less salient, and this has consequences for clustering. For example, a famous 1952 paper by the sociologist Ruby Kennedy collected almost a century of marriage records in New Haven, Connecticut. Among the oldest records dating from 1870, virtually 100 percent of Italians, Poles, and Irish married exclusively within their own groups.[17] By 2015, in contrast, around 40 percent of U.S. marriages were to people who were not even from the same religion.[18]

The advantages and limitations of using estimated ancestry proportions in lieu of self-defined race are well described in the scientific literature. With ancestry inferred from DNA, multiracial individuals are no longer forced into a single classification, and one avoids the messy and awkward problem of self-report. But the process of defining the reference samples is still subjective because these samples are drawn from living individuals, not the hypothetical ancestral populations they are meant to proxy for. These latent ancestral populations must also be arbitrarily bounded in time; otherwise, all humans would simply be Africans. We must also allow that pre-Columbian populations were not all static and reproductively isolated.[19] Despite these profound drawbacks, this approach of inferring ancestry from DNA is now standard in genetic studies to avoid the kind of confounding labeled as "population stratification." Importantly, it is intended only to address genetic confounding, not any of the sociological mechanisms that operate through racism and other forms of differential treatment.

Most genetic variation is within group and not between groups. To illustrate this concept, take any human trait, such as a disease. Consider Parkinson's disease, for example, a neurodegenerative condition that causes rigidity and difficulty with movement and balance. The causes are still largely unknown, and globally about 1 percent of those over age sixty are affected. Because the disease exists in every human population, almost all the variation that exists is between people with and without Parkinson's within any given region. At the same time, there are slight variations from place to place, with North Americans having an age-adjusted incidence rate of over 20 per 1,000 per year, whereas that number is around 15 in Australasia and East Asia, 12 in Latin America, and 8 in sub-Saharan Africa.[20] This is the same pattern that holds for almost all genetic variations: they exist in every population but at slightly different prevalences, such that almost all the variation that exists within humanity exists within every group of reasonable size.

A consequence of this pattern is that ancestries are not especially informative about risk of disease or other traits, except to the extent that they are correlated with sociological mechanisms for historical reasons, like the slave trade. Previously enslaved North Americans were not chosen randomly from around the world but instead were drawn primarily from West Africa. This means that whatever long-term consequences of this social history still reverberate will be concentrated in that ancestry group but not because of any biological difference. Therefore, the use of genetic ancestry in place of race risks profound measurement error when the salient etiologic mechanism does not operate through a purely genetic pathway. Although its common application in genetic epidemiology might be defensible, its spillover into population epidemiology is probably not. Moreover, the assignment of race as a latent ancestry cluster is not necessarily concordant with assignment by self-identification because the latter accounts for affiliations and experiences that are irrelevant to the statistical analysis of DNA markers.

Wayne Joseph was a high school principal in Chino, California, when he took a recreational DNA test in 2003. His family had emigrated from southern Louisiana, and he had a solidly Black American identity rooted in the historical segregation of that region. His story of self-discovery, told eloquently in a 2003 essay in the magazine *LA Weekly* by the journalist Erin Aubrey Kaplan, began when the DNA test results came back with the news that Joseph had 0 percent African ancestry.[21] The "one-drop rule" is the long-standing social convention in the United States that ties Black identity to even the slightest evident degree of African ancestry. But Joseph's DNA result, reported without any margin of error or other admission of uncertainty, denied him even that one drop. Kaplan's essay outlines the struggle to reconcile the supposed objectivity of DNA with Joseph's lifetime of experiences, affiliations, and cultural attitudes that all define identity in ways that cannot be undone. Forced to pick a single truth from these two conflicting versions of who he was, Joseph ultimately decided that he already knew perfectly well who he was and was too old to change his mind about it. Self-identity, to him, was the true definition of race. It was the DNA test that was in error, not the other way around.

Ultimately, estimated ancestry proportions from DNA are strictly hypothetical constructs from a mathematical procedure and have no common-sense interpretations as races or ethnicities, whether sociological or biological. For example, Joseph's DNA ancestry test reported that he was 39 percent Native American. What does it even mean for one to have 39 percent Native American ancestry? Is that number supposed to imply that 39 percent of all of one's ancestors were Native Americans? Thirty-nine out of every one hundred ancestors sounds like a very precise proportion. But how many ancestors does a person actually have? For example, we now believe that non-Africans typically have about 2 percent Neanderthal ancestry based on comparison of variants with ancient DNA. But the last contact between Neanderthals and *Homo sapiens* was more than thirty or forty thousand years ago. Just going back one thousand years to around the Battle of Hastings, we each have around 2^{30} ancestors, which is more than a billion people, far more than the number of people alive on earth one thousand years ago. Clearly this ancestry proportion is a completely imaginary number. Its true value can't be observed, even hypothetically, and therefore, no assertion about its value can be objectively refuted. This is also why recreational ancestry companies have such an iron-clad business model because they provide information that can never be refuted, even though competing companies can provide wildly different estimates. [22] Thus, when considering misclassification of race or ethnicity, ancestry testing can never hope to serve as any kind of gold standard measure in the way that, say, a blood test for malaria can.

Much of this book is devoted to statistical adjustments made to observed racial and ethnic disparities and the inadvertent harm that these adjustments often cause when researchers are careless or misguided. In the case of measurement, however, trying to account for misclassifications of race and ethnicity, the problem is that adjustments for this impropriety are *not* made, nor could they ever be done so. There are standard adjustment procedures for measurement error in the statistics literature, but these are based on validation studies and the resulting sensitivities and specificities that can be estimated from those studies. [23] As discussed earlier, there can be no gold standard measure for race and ethnicity because these are states of self-identity and not subject to verification or refutation. "If you cannot measure it, you cannot improve it," wrote Lord Kelvin.[24] This is exactly what makes race and ethnicity unsuitable for applications in science and medicine; they cannot be measured objectively and thus cannot be improved.

If one focuses on differential social treatment (i.e., racism) as the mechanism underlying racial disparities in health or economic outcomes, then one could opt for racial classification by external observers as the one that is more salient than the person's own self-identity. This is the logic behind the idea of *street race*, a term coined by the sociologist Nancy López.[25] In this framework, it is important to record not only how individuals classify themselves but also how others would classify them if, for instance, they saw them walking down the street. Not only are these two forms of identity both potentially relevant in their own ways, but a discrepancy between them is an indication of a person who will experience some tension between their self-awareness and their social experiences. Other scholars, like the sociologist Aliya Saperstein, study the distinct factors shaping each of these dimensions and how they affect each other. For example, people perceived by others as Hispanic were more likely to experience material hardship, and people who evidenced material hardship were more likely to be perceived as Hispanic, regardless of their actual self-identity.[26] Likewise, odds of being arrested by the police were nearly three times higher for people who were classified by others as Black, even if they did not identify themselves as Black, whereas there was no increase in the odds of being arrested among those self-identifying as Black if they were not seen by others as Black.[27] The suspicion that race perceived by others may be the more salient factor in attracting the attention of law enforcement is further supported by the finding that Black motorists are stopped more than white motorists during the daytime but that this racial discrepancy disappears under the cover of darkness.[28]

DNA-based ancestry testing does not define a person's race, as explained earlier. But in the era in which such testing has become commonplace, it can influence how people self-identify. This makes perfect sense. For the test result to change someone's self-identity, it is not necessary that it be an accurate indication of their "true race," only that the person believes that it is. We saw in the case of Wayne Joseph that he rejected the test result in favor of his lived experiences. Something similar happened in the cases of white supremacists who took the ancestry test in the previous decade to confirm their racial purity, only to reject the test if it yielded any ambiguous results.[29] And yet it has also been observed that people who receive ancestry test results are more likely to redefine themselves as multiracial.[30] Then of course there are the more cynical uses of such tests. The legal scholar David Bernstein recounts the story of Ralph Taylor, a businessman who had spent his entire life as a white man but who successfully applied for his insurance company to be classified as a "minority business enterprise" based on an ancestry test that reported him to be 4 percent sub-Saharan African.[31] Another infamous example of using ancestry testing to support a tenuous claims of racial identity is that of Senator Elizabeth Warren, who in 2020 used such a result in a somewhat less successful attempt to bolster her claim of Native American heritage.[32]

The absence of any objective definition for the boundaries of a racial group also has implications for issues of representativeness and generalizability. A published study may make inference about the prevalence of some trait or the effect of some exposure in Blacks versus whites, based on a study population self-classifying into each group, but with no assurance that these participants are informative about others in that wider population. The scholarly literature is replete with these dubious generalizations. In a typical example of this kind of research paper, the dermatologist Mathew Birnbaum and colleagues recently collected microscopic photographs of the scalps of ninety-nine Hispanics, forty-four African Americans, and twenty-three Caucasians recruited at a New York City hospital in an effort to determine which was the most hirsute race.[33] The Caucasians were significantly more hairy, in case you're curious. But the more important point is this: Why should we think that these twenty-three Caucasians are informative about all white people? The reflexive leap from what is observed in this handful of white people to what is presumed to be known about white people in general seems absurd. And yet it is one of the most common inferences in fields like psychology and medicine, where random sampling from enumerated populations is not the norm.

This inferential leap is problematic in part because there is no unambiguous denominator population from which such a sample would be drawn, even if the authors wished to do so. The identities present in the modern American context may be rooted in ancestries, but these ancestral populations do not share that identity. For example, a person of Chinese ancestry in the United States may be taught to classify themselves as "Asian" according to the current census categories, but a person of Chinese ancestry in China would not. They would instead be ethnically Zhuang, Hui, Han, Manchu, and so forth, or perhaps, in a more cosmopolitan and nationalistic sense, simply Chinese, but never "Asian." Likewise, there are no Hispanics outside of the United States, only Mexicans and Bolivians and so on, or indigenous ethnic identities like Aymara or Guarani that were completely excluded from the official Office of Management and Budget Directive 15 definitions used in the United States until 2024. A more cohesive African American identity was formed only by the relentless cultural violence of severing people from their original identities and languages such as Yoruba, Kongo, or Ewe, the living descendants of whom do not identify as "Black" except to the extent that they have learned to do so as an American cultural export.

This cultural particularism is evidenced by the wide variation in how racial and ethnic terms are reported in the scientific literature. Taking several leading medical and epidemiological journals as a case study, Erika Lynn-Green and colleagues recently reported that studies with U.S. authors were dramatically more likely to report race or ethnicity of participants (73 percent and 47 percent of papers, respectively) than authors from other countries (26 percent and 14 percent, respectively).[34] The consequence for science is a racial Tower of Babel, in which race-specific knowledge generated in one place has no unambiguous application elsewhere. How can modern research hope to flourish in a global scientific community if the categories used do not transport beyond the boundaries of local custom? A compelling example of this dilemma is the story of clinical estimation of kidney function. Physicians need to be able to check how a patient's kidneys are working for a variety of reasons, including safe dosage of medication. But direct measurement of kidneys filtering a patient's blood would be invasive, expensive, and time-consuming. To solve this problem, researchers developed equations in the 1970s to estimate clearance of blood through the kidneys simply as a function of a patient's sex, weight, age, and serum creatinine.[35]

In 1999, the nephrologist Andrew Levey and colleagues proposed a new and improved equation for this purpose based on analysis of around thirteen hundred white and two hundred Black volunteers with kidney disease who had enrolled in a dietary intervention study in the early 1990s. The authors fit a regression model to the data, predicting kidney function in relation to variables available in the dataset, and noticed that self-identified Black race was a "significant" predictor in this model.[36] Therefore, their new prediction equation, called the MDRD equation (after the acronym of the original dietary intervention study), included sex, age, race (Black or white), and serum creatinine. The race term inflates the estimated kidney function score by about 20 percent for Blacks.[37] Interestingly, these authors deleted weight from their model, instead setting the model to assume that the patient was 170 centimeters tall and weighed 63 kilograms. This new approach was widely adopted around the world, but it presents a dilemma of how to interpret the race variable. Did the roughly two hundred Black Americans who volunteered for the diet trial represent Black Americans or all Black people in the world? Most labs around the world simply generated both a Black and a non-Black estimate and left this decision to the medical provider. Attempts to replicate the necessity of a race correction in other Black populations in Africa, Europe, and Brazil generally failed.[38] This led some guidelines to interpret the correction as specific to Black Americans and therefore that other Blacks in the world should be provided with the white estimate. For example, the French Haute Autorité de Santé advised in 2011 that because the estimates were derived from Black Americans, the race correction should not be applied to French Blacks.[39] Despite this advice, it is easy to find online kidney function calculators in France that have a checkbox for *peau noire* (black skin).[40]

It is no surprise that these ambiguities over definitions of race and racial cut-off points for disease have pervasive impacts on research meant to study disparities. In a typical example, Priya Vart and colleagues studied trial data to assess the effectiveness and safety of dapagliflozin in Black and white patients from North and South America.[41] This drug is a sodium-glucose cotransporter-2 inhibitor commonly used to treat diabetes and slow the progression of kidney failure among those diagnosed with chronic kidney disease. The researchers wanted to know if the drug worked the same way in Black and white patients with chronic kidney disease, so they used data on nearly two hundred self-described Black and nearly eleven hundred self-described white patients from a large randomized trial conducted in multiple countries in North and South America. Inclusion in the trial was premised on a specific range of values for the glomerular filtration rate, but this was assessed using the "race-corrected" formula discussed earlier. What are the measurement error implications of assuming that "Black" and "white" self-definitions are the same across countries of North and South America and then restricting the analysis to those with kidney disease as defined by race-specific criteria that were derived in North American populations?

I'll discuss the kidney function score example in greater detail in chapter 7, but the point here is that race in this kind of medical application is inadmissible because it is completely contextual—it has no consistency from one place or time to the next. The scientific foundations of medicine are premised on measurement and validation, and there is no possibility of this in the case of race. It just so happened that the United States became the dominant producer and exporter of biomedical and scientific knowledge after World War II, and it just so happened that America at this time had an apartheid social system that classified citizens according to an idiosyncratic racial hierarchy that persisted from the period of chattel slavery. Imagine if history had played out differently and it was India that became the world's dominant research engine, and they made their kidney function equation based on caste, with a correction factor for Dalits. This thought experiment might provide some hint of how strange America's race obsession can seem to the rest of the world. Notice also that the creators of the new kidney function equation dropped weight from their model so that they could make room for race. It was easier for them to assume that all people weighed 63 kilograms than it was to assume that Black and white kidneys might work the same way.

CHAPTER VII

Proxies and Predictions

T he population of New York State in 1990 was just under eighteen million people, and over the next decade, this number grew
steadily.[1] Plotting these numbers with the population on the vertical axis and the year on the horizontal axis reveals a clear pattern of linear
growth (figure 7.1).

If asked to predict the 2001 population from this historical pattern, most
people would reason that the population changed by a million people over
the eleven years plotted here (1990–2000), and so the average annual change
was 1 million/11 = 91,000 people. Therefore, the 2001 population could be
predicted to be about 19.09 million, and in fact, it was. This is a simple linear
regression model, the workhorse of modern social and biomedical sciences.
Under the assumption that the world is made up of straight lines, we can
specify a mathematical function that fits such a trend through the observed
data points. In this case, that mathematical function would be that the current
population = baseline population + (90,000 × change in years). Population
growth isn't always so predictably linear, especially over longer periods of
time, and one might model percentage growth as linear rather than absolute
growth. But my point is to convey the idea of a regression model because it
plays such a central role in quantitative social and biological sciences. I have
mentioned regression models already several times in the previous chapters,
and they are often used for the kinds of adjustments discussed earlier, such
as for confounding factors. Putting race and some covariate together in a

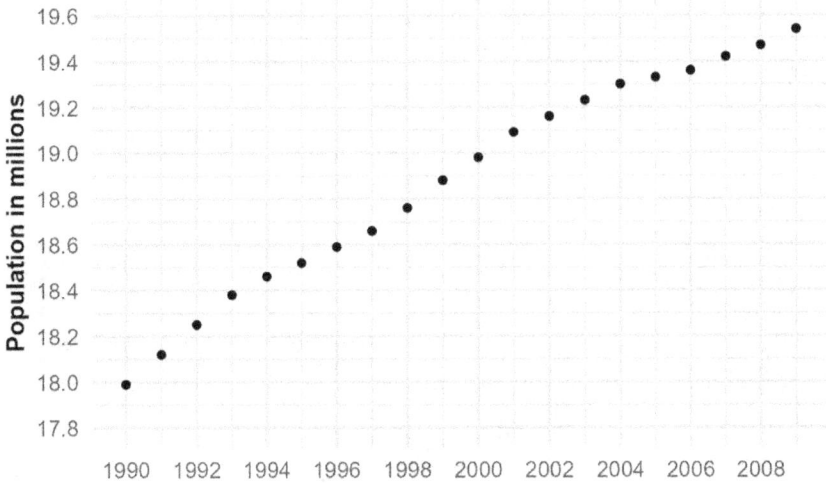

Figure 7.1 Population of New York State by year.

regression model changes the interpretation of the race term to be conditional on the other quantity, essentially holding it constant.

For example, if I had a model for the race disparity in the effect of treatment (X) on some outcome (Y), the linear model would be written as Average Y $= \beta_0 + \beta_1 X + \beta_2$ Race. Greek letters like β (beta) are used to represent things that are estimated, whereas Roman letters like Y, X, and "Race" are used for information that is already present in the dataset. Specifically, β_1 and β_2 are slope coefficients, meaning that they represent the estimated change in Y per unit change in a variable in the dataset; β_1 shows how Y changes with a change in X, holding Race constant, and β_2 shows how Y changes with a change in Race, holding X constant.

The additivity of the model (plus signs between the terms) implies that the X effect is constant across race groups and the race gap is constant at every level of treatment X. The lines for the change in the average outcome at each level of treatment are parallel, always separated by a distance of β_2, the race gap. One can interpret this gap as X-adjusted because X is in this model alongside race, and so we fix X at a single value to interpret β_2, but it doesn't matter at what level this is fixed because β_2 is constant across all values of X (figure 7.2). That might seem suspicious, and indeed, many people question these simplistic constancy assumptions.[2] There are ways to

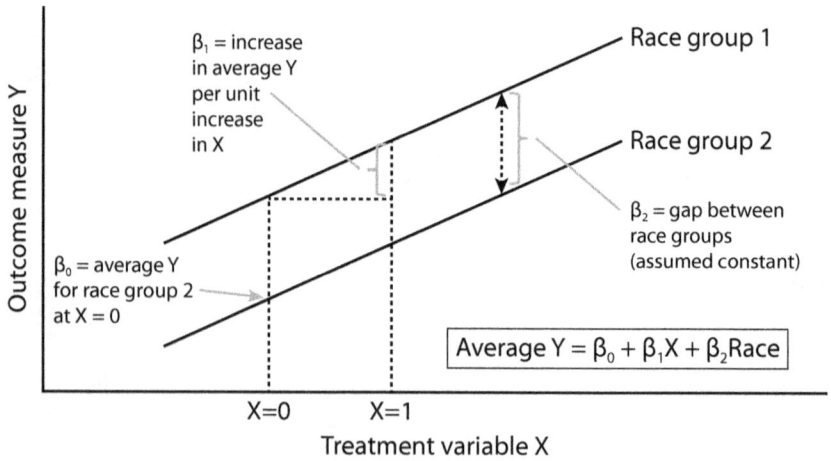

Figure 7.2 Schematic representation of a linear regression model of two race groups in relation to exposure X.

relax these assumptions by making the models more complex, like adding interaction terms, but regression in one form or another remains the standard approach in the vast majority of published studies.

As an example, suppose that a researcher modeled systolic blood pressure (SBP), measured in millimeters of mercury (mmHg), in Black and white men in relation to sodium consumption (NaCl) estimated from a twenty-four-hour diet recall and measured in grams per day. The variable Black takes the value of 1 for Black men and takes the value of 0 for white men. Then the regression model would be SBP = β_0 + β_1NaCl + β_2Black (figure 7.3).

In this equation, β_0 represents the blood pressure for white men who have zero sodium consumption, but this is unlikely to be observed in the dataset because everyone gets at least some sodium in their diet. The β_1 term encodes the increase in blood pressure for each one-gram increase of sodium intake, and this applies to both race groups because the lines are parallel. Finally, the β_2 term provides the (constant) blood pressure gap between Black and white men at every level of sodium intake. A classic disparities analysis might involve conducting a null-hypothesis significance test (chapter 8) of the β_2 term to see if it is "significantly" greater than zero. If it is, the investigator might state that there is a "significant" racial disparity, even while holding sodium consumption constant. If other variables were

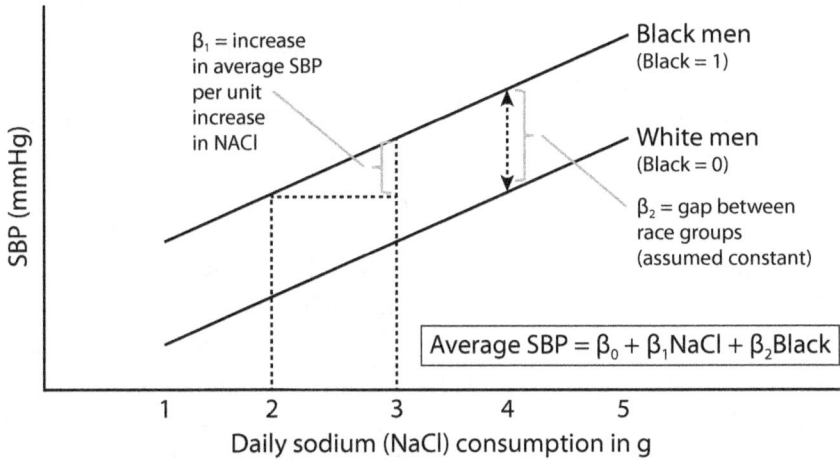

β_1 = increase in average SBP per unit increase in NACl

Black men (Black = 1)

White men (Black = 0)

β_2 = gap between race groups (assumed constant)

Average SBP = $\beta_0 + \beta_1$NaCl + β_2Black

SBP (mmHg)

Daily sodium (NaCl) consumption in g

Figure 7.3 Schematic representation of a linear regression model of systolic blood pressure among Black and white men in relation to sodium consumption.

added to the regression models with their own coefficients, then these factors would also be "held constant" in the model.

There are many uses for regression models, but primarily they serve the main functions of data analysis outlined in chapter 2, namely description, prediction, and causal inference. For description, the fitted linear trend smooths over noise in the data series. One may visualize a cloud of points from which the trend is not evident, but the regression model finds the best-fitting line through the data points and reveals a smooth tendency.[3] Prediction is easily understood from our earlier example using the New York State population series. With a trend line fit for 1990 to 2000, we were able to extrapolate this line to the next year to predict its expected value if the same trend continued. Finally, for causal inference, regression models are very useful for holding covariates constant, as in the earlier example with racial differences in blood pressure in relation to sodium consumption. This is a way of comparing people with similar characteristics or exposures, as we would do if we matched people in the study design or in the analysis. There are many flavors of regression model, including logistic regression for categorical outcomes and proportional hazards regression for survival time analyses, and these express parallelism on different mathematical scales (see chapter 9). But despite all the many variations and options, they are all essentially just ways of plotting the average outcome at each value of an exposure or predictor, often while holding constant the influences of other variables that are considered to be a nuisance, like confounders.

The focus in this chapter is on prediction and the potential role of race and ethnicity in various predictive algorithms. Such predictions are generally facilitated with regression models as described earlier, which is why it was necessary to explain them at the start. So then let's return to the prediction of kidney function that was introduced in the last chapter, the estimated glomerular filtration rate (eGFR).[4] In the 1990s when Andrew Levey and colleagues sought to develop a new predictive equation for estimating kidney function from serum creatinine and a few other clinical variables, they employed a dataset in which they had a gold standard outcome measure, a laborious clinical assessment of true kidney function, and they modeled this as the outcome of a regression equation, using creatine and the other variables as the predictors. They found race had an influence on the estimated kidney function score, and on this statistical basis, it was included in the new prediction equation.[5]

We have already discussed the concern that the small number of self-identified Black participants in this study were serving as proxies for all Black people and that these participants were volunteers with kidney disease, so hardly representative in any sense. In fact, Levey et al. improved on this equation in 2009 with new estimates from a more flexible model, based on more than twelve thousand participants with and without kidney disease, and in the new model, the race coefficient was reduced in magnitude but still present.[6] But why should race modify the relationship between serum creatinine and kidney function? There is no way to know based on the data used for these predictions. The participants in the studies could be unusual in some way, or the population of Blacks in the United States might truly differ from other populations in any number of relevant social, material, and lifestyle dimensions that affect kidney function.

Levey and colleagues included in their paper only one post hoc explanation to justify adding a racial adjustment, rationalizing that "on average, Black persons have greater muscle mass than white persons."[7] Muscle mass is relevant here because serum creatinine is a by-product of muscle metabolism, and so more muscle means more creatinine. To support this curious assertion, they cited three obscure papers, all of which relied on small unrepresentative convenience samples and with obvious socioeconomic confounding. The first was an observation from a laboratory in Upton, New

York, from the 1970s, where the authors recruited and measured around fifty Black men and women who were staff at the facility or their friends and family.[8] The second study examined about 250 volunteer children from Bogalusa, Louisiana, in the mid-1970s.[9] And the third included thirty Black and thirty white subjects recruited from the medical, nursing, laboratory, portering, and domestic staff of a British hospital.[10] One can easily guess that the less muscular medical staff were more likely found among the thirty whites and the more muscular portering and domestic staff among the thirty Blacks, raising some doubts about what this might really tell us about population patterns of musculature.

Even if these studies were representative and valid, differences in the means of a trait between groups are unlikely to be clinically relevant for the prediction score. This use of race as a proxy for an unmeasured quantity like muscle mass arises from a common statistical fallacy: the conflation of "significant" prediction of the average value using a regression model with meaningful prediction for an individual from the population. The average value of a trait may differ between race groups, but the vast majority of the individuals in the population do not sit at the average value. Every trait has some continuous distribution in a population. Take a trait like height, which will exhibit a bell-shaped distribution around the group average. When lined up by increasing height, there will be a spread in the values, from very short people on the left to very tall people on the right.

For example, the average height of Japanese men is 1.7 meters and the average height of Japanese women is 1.6 meters, so these averages are different, and many people would feel comfortable asserting that men are taller than women in Japan (figure 7.4).

But in Japan, not all men are 1.7 meters tall. In fact, very few men are exactly 1.7 meters. Rather, 95 percent of men fall in a range between roughly 1.5 and 1.9 meters. Likewise, 95 percent of women fall in a range between roughly 1.4 and 1.8 meters. This means that although it is a true statement that the *average* Japanese man is taller than the *average* Japanese woman, it is also true that many women are taller than many men. Indeed, a Japanese person with a height of 1.65 meters is equally likely to be male or female. Whenever the spread of values around the average, which is called the *variance*, is large with respect to the difference between the averages, the group indicator will be a poor predictor for any individual. Use of race as a "significant" predictor in statistical models is almost always invalidated by this simple relationship.[11]

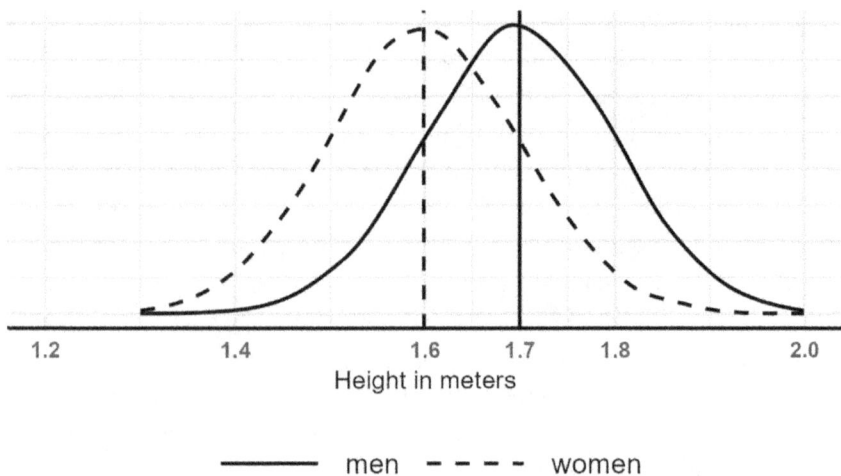

Figure 7.4 The distributions of heights of Japanese men and women in meters.

What is the actual relationship between race and muscle mass in the United States? Curiously, I didn't find any publication addressing this question directly using population-representative data, but it is easy to look in such a dataset to find the answer. The U.S. National Center for Health Statistics conducts an annual examination survey of American adults and children with interviews, physical examinations, and laboratory tests, including dual-energy x-ray absorptiometry (DXA) for estimation of muscle mass (technically, lean mass, but most of the variation in lean mass is muscle). So, I simply fit some very simple linear regression models predicting continuous lean mass as estimated by DXA in the 2013–2014 National Health and Nutrition Examination Survey dataset, using population-weighted samples of self-identified non–Hispanic Black and white adults aged nineteen and older.[12]

A simple measure of the total variation in the outcome that is explained by a predictor in a linear regression model is the so-called model R^2, which ranges from none (0 percent) to all (100 percent) of the variation explained. If 100 percent of the variation is explained, then if I know the predictor, I know the exact value of the outcome. For instance, if you know someone's height in centimeters and you want to predict the height in inches, then that model will have $R^2 = 100$ percent because one inch is equivalent to

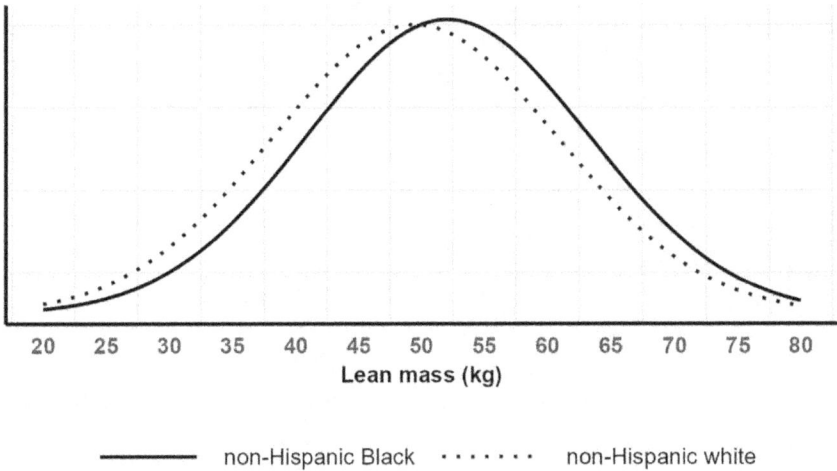

Figure 7.5 Non-Hispanic white versus non-Hispanic Black lean mass from dual X-ray absorptiometry.

2.54 centimeters with no residual error. In contrast, predicting a person's height as a function of their parents' height gives an R^2 of about 0.36.[13] Finally, predicting a person's height as a function of their favorite color gives an R^2 of zero.

The R^2 for the prediction of lean mass as a function of Black or white race is only about 1 percent, which is to say, almost nothing (figure 7.5).

If I add sex to the model, the R^2 jumps up from 1 percent to 53 percent, with sex obviously accounting for almost all of that predictive power (figure 7.6).

To get a sense of how small this race contribution to prediction really is, I must compare it to other binary variables that one could use instead to predict lean mass. A common measure of obesity is the body mass index (BMI), which is defined as weight (in kilograms) divided by the square of height (in meters). The dividing line between the top half of values and the bottom half of values in a dataset is referred to as the *median* value. Predicting lean mass with a median split of BMI (at 27.1 kg/m^2) gives an R^2 of 14 percent. Adding sex to that model brings it up to 67 percent (figure 7.7). BMI includes both height and weight, but even ignoring weight, predicting lean mass with a median split of height (at 1.67 meters) gives an R^2 of

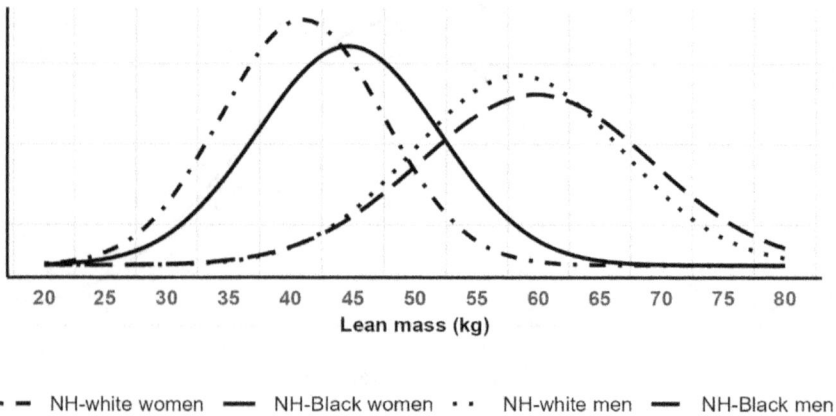

Figure 7.6 Non-Hispanic white versus non-Hispanic Black men and women lean mass from dual X-ray absorptiometry.

44 percent. One could refine this further, perhaps by age adjusting or making separate models by sex, but the basic result is clear: any differences in average muscle mass *between* race groups are tiny compared to the variation *within* each race group. That means that race lacks utility for individual prediction of this trait.[14] If Levey and colleagues had really needed a convenient proxy for muscle mass, they would have been much better off using height, weight, or some combination of those variables.

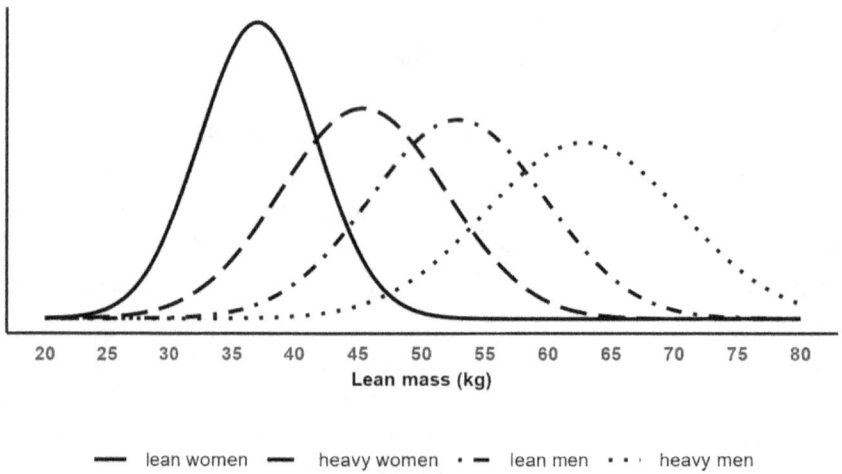

— lean women — heavy women • — lean men • • • heavy men

Figure 7.7 Lean and heavy men and women, lean mass from dual X-ray absorptiometry.

Race was in fact a significant predictor of average kidney function in the datasets analyzed by Levey and colleagues, even though this was clearly not because it was serving as a proxy for muscle mass. More likely it stood in for any of a large number of social and environmental determinants of kidney function, including physical activity and diet, arising as functions of social class, occupation, neighborhood, and other behavioral and cultural factors that cannot be expected to be stable over time or place.[15] It's no wonder, therefore, that this race "correction" could not be replicated in datasets from outside of the United States.[16] A joint task force of the American Society of Nephrology and the National Kidney Foundation finally called for an end to this race correction in 2021,[17] but many labs are not yet caught up to the new recommendations and therefore are still adjusting up Black eGFR estimates by 16 to 21 percent. This makes it more difficult for Black patients to qualify for transplants and other treatment interventions, requiring them to have more advanced disease than a patient who is not Black to achieve the same eGFR value.[18]

There are many similar examples in which race or ethnicity works its way into prediction equations in medicine, criminal justice, economics, and other fields. There is no doubt that profound racial and ethnic stratification exists in many societies, so that finding these categories to be predictive of a wide range of outcomes is no surprise. But as the previous example highlights, prediction of an average value within a population is very different from prediction of an individual's value.[19] If the variation within a population is small relative to the difference in the averages, then individual prediction could in principle be valid. However, if variation within a population is large relative to the difference in the averages, then individual prediction becomes hopeless.

Consider examples of both those scenarios. The annual base salary for journalists in the United States is roughly $30,000 to $50,000, whereas the annual base salary for plastic surgeons is roughly $300,000 to $500,000. This is a setting in which the between-group difference is large relative to the within-group difference, and so group membership will be highly informative for individual prediction. This implies that knowing which group a person is from will change one's predicted income for that individual dramatically. Almost every single plastic surgeon makes more money than almost every single journalist. For the opposite extreme, consider that the mean age of Japanese people is forty-seven years old and the mean age of Canadians is forty-two years. So Japanese are on average significantly older than

Canadians. But this information is almost completely useless in guessing the age of a random person drawn from one of these populations. This implies that when you try to guess a random person's age, the magnitude of your error will decrease negligibly if you know which country the person is from.

There are a handful of real examples where race and ethnicity can be sufficiently informative to support individual-level prediction because the trait distributions are so disparate. For example, we define wealth as assets, such as investments, savings in the bank, and the value of one's property. The racial disparity in wealth in the United States is so extreme that it is highly informative for individual prediction. The median household wealth in 2019 was $206,400 for Asians, $187,300 for non-Hispanic whites, $31,700 for Hispanics, and $14,100 for Blacks.[20] In clinical medicine, by contrast, there is almost no physical trait besides skin color that is sufficiently disparate to support individual prediction. However, this hasn't stopped clinical medicine from using race and ethnicity in all sorts of predictive equations and treatment algorithms.[21]

A compelling example of unjustified use of race as a proxy for an unmeasured variable in a model is the recent case of "race norming" by the National Football League (NFL). This was the practice of assuming a lower baseline cognitive ability for Black athletes in settling compensation claims for concussion-related injuries. Chronic traumatic encephalopathy (CTE) is a brain condition precipitated by repeated blows to the head, such as what occurs in the daily life of a professional football player. Because this was a routine occupational hazard of NFL employment, the league reached a legal settlement in 2015 that required those who claimed work-related injury to undergo cognitive evaluation, the results of which determined the amount of compensation they would receive, if any. The problem was that claimants needed to show that they had lost cognitive function but they had no baseline evaluations from which to estimate a decline. The test score results were therefore "normed" to the demographic characteristics of the player, most importantly age, educational attainment, and race. The ostensible aim was to evaluate the player's cognitive function in relation to a referent population, and Black players, who composed more than two-thirds of NFL players, were presumed in the algorithm to have lower baseline cognitive function in the general population. Because a Black player at a given age and educational level was assumed to start with less cognitive function than a comparable white player, it was more difficult for the Black player to demonstrate a deficit and, therefore, more difficult to collect compensation.[22]

The NFL at first defended the race-norming approach as being fairer to the players by accounting for their demographic differences but eventually succumbed to a tsunami of criticism and lawsuits. They finally abandoned the practice in the summer of 2021.[23] There are many problems evident in this ill-fated policy, starting with the presumption of inherent racial inferiority that ignores differences in enriched environments, educational quality, and other social determinants of cognitive test results, some of which are intergenerational.[24] Another theme is the one that was stressed in the previous eGFR example, which is that a model about a population average is not necessarily applicable to an individual prediction. To assign everyone the average value of their demographic group, which is essentially what race norming in this context does, is to engage in crude stereotyping. It's contrary to the individual justice that these people seek in compensation claims. Suppose you go to court because your bank has robbed you of a million dollars and the judge tells you that, because the average person only has $50,000 in their account, that is the number they'll assume you have lost.

There is an even more insidious injustice going on, which is the presumption on the part of the algorithm designers that they are entitled to select the salient factors upon which the group average for an individual is to be determined. Age and educational attainment are reasonably objective determinants of cognition, and so it seems obvious to use them, but why should the next most salient feature of a person's identity necessarily be race? After all, an individual can have many identities, and maybe it is more relevant that they are Catholic, or from Alabama, or foreign born, or an only child, or something else. Most other countries in the world would never do as the United States and presume that race is the primary, reflexive, all-purpose demographic affiliation for all its citizens.

Writing about this phenomenon as an ethical consideration more than a decade ago, I expressed the concern that when individuals' unknown values are imputed from their group averages, the statistical procedure risks serving as "the handmaiden of existing prejudices."[25] The common algorithmic use of race in prediction is premised on leveraging informative markers. But perhaps this is merely a self-fulfilling prophecy that bins people according to a folkloric taxonomy and then blithely perpetuates this same taxonomy on the argument that it is informative to do so. Many common statistical procedures are based on investigator-specified groupings, including multilevel (hierarchical) modeling, which intentionally biases estimates toward group averages to improve prediction.[26] This routine statistical grouping has a mathematical justification, but it also facilitates the admission of social conventions and prejudices into the analytic process, and this can have important ramifications for the predicted values for individuals within the population, as in the NFL example described earlier.

Here is another statistical application that helps explain what I mean about how socially defined categories can launder existing prejudices into the semblance of statistical objectivity. Consider performance on an academic test for schoolchildren. Suppose that every student has a latent (that is, unobserved) score that reflects their intrinsic talent and knowledge, and the observed test score reveals a randomly noisy estimate of that true value. This implies that the true value could be higher or lower than the measured value because the error is random. Because of this random error, if the test is given to a whole classroom of students, then the child with the highest score most likely got a little bit lucky and scored above their true ability, whereas the child with the lowest score most likely got a little bit unlucky and scored below their true ability. This means that if tested again, the highest-scoring student is expected to score lower than the first time and the lowest-scoring student is expected to score higher. This is a general phenomenon known as "regression to the mean."[27] In fact, this is how intentionally biased statistical procedures like multilevel modeling are justified because "shrinking" the extreme scores toward the average of all students tends to improve prediction through this same logic.

But students might not only belong to the classroom as a whole; there might also be distinct subpopulations with distinct average abilities. Suppose that the classroom average test score is 100, but it is composed of an equal number of boys and girls, and the boys have an average test score of 90, whereas girls have an average of 110. When a student gets a test score of 100, this is a valid estimate of that student's true latent score. But we can do better. If the student is a girl, we can bet that her true score will lie between 100 and 110, and if the student is a boy, we can bet that his score will lie between 90 and 100. If we bet in this way, we are *guaranteed* (at the level of the classroom as a whole) to outperform the predictions of someone simply using the observed scores alone without incorporating information on the gender of the student.[28] This technique is referred to as *shrinkage*, and the analyst who doesn't shrink the results in this way is essentially ignoring important information. It seems obvious that one can't predict better by ignoring some important information.

The unavoidable ethical dilemma lies in the fact that we (the analysts) get to decide what constitutes a subgroup and to which subgroup each person belongs. Let's continue the example above. The boys have an average score of 90 and the girls an average score of 110. Now suppose that average scores for Blacks and whites in the classroom are also 90 and 110, respectively. One student, a Black girl named Celia, takes the test and scores 100 points. If we decide that the groups of greatest interest to us are boys and girls, we would bump up Celia's score to a higher value because she is a girl, and in aggregate (across all the students in the class), we are *guaranteed* to do better in our predictions compared to someone who uses only the raw scores. However, if we decide that the groups of interest to us are Blacks and whites, we would reduce Celia's score because she is Black and our ensemble predictions would still outperform someone using the raw scores. We are guaranteed to win either way, in the sense of reducing our prediction error, and so choosing gender or race as the salient grouping is of little concern to us. But it makes a big difference to Celia, whose corrected score is pushed up or down depending on whether we prioritize her gender or her race as the salient marker of academic ability.

One natural question might be: Why choose? Why not use all possible groups? Obviously, there are some practical limitations to slicing the population so finely that most cells become sparse or even empty. But this is indeed one current approach of quantitative intersectionality researchers, who seek to use these shrinkage techniques to simultaneously consider many important axes of identity simultaneously.[29] Nonetheless, what is much more common in practice is to respect parsimony by using only a small number of selected factors as most informative, especially age, sex, and (particularly in the United States) race, as in the case of the kidney function score discussed earlier. Think of the standard American clinical presentation of a medical patient as, say, "a fifty-three-year-old Black male," as though these are the three dimensions that form the most important aspects of identity for physicians.[30] Another natural question is whether we even care about the individual prediction if the goal of shrinkage is to guarantee an improved ensemble performance, which means a reduced error across the whole sample population. This next story provides a real-life example of shrinking scores up or down to show how consequential this phenomenon can be to the individual.

The Educational Testing Service (ETS) is a private nonprofit American company that develops standardized tests for high school students, including those commonly taken by high school students to qualify for university admissions. The ETS devised a program in the 1990s in which high-performing students from predominantly low-income schools were designated "Strivers" and their university admissions test scores were augmented because they performed well even under adverse social and material conditions.[31] "It stands to reason," wrote two noted sociologists at the time, "that a student from a materially and educationally impoverished environment who does fairly well on the [test] and better than other students who come from a similar environment is probably stronger than the unadjusted score indicates."[32] Anthony Carnevale, vice president of ETS, made a similar argument in favor of augmenting the scores: "When you look at a Striver who gets a score of 1000, you're looking at someone who really performs at 1200."[33]

Considering regression to the mean, however, the achieved scores of the "Strivers" might instead be better predicted to be overestimates of their true abilities, suggesting that instead of bumping their scores up, a more accurate measure might be achieved by penalizing them and shrinking their scores back closer to the averages of their groups.[34] With this reasoning, a dissenting ETS statistician named Howard Wainer argued against the proposed program and instead for shrinkage to the group mean: "When you look at a Striver who gets a score of 1000, you're probably looking at someone who really performs at 950. And, alas, a Striver is probably weaker than the unadjusted score indicates."[35] In the end, the "Striver" program was abandoned without ever being widely implemented, although it seems that pressure on the ETS to ditch the program was more about the politics than the statistics.[36]

Most people imagine that statistical tasks like prediction are objective, mathematical exercises, but as seen in this example, whether one should adjust a student's score up or down depends just as much on the mental model one chooses for the meaning of group membership.[37] If the minority or low-income school is a handicap like hanging an extra weight around the student's neck before they run a race, then the score adjusted upward will be the better predictor of a future performance when the weight is removed. However, if the average score from a minority or low-income school is the best representation of the aggregate tendency of students from this environment, then adjusting a high score by lowering it closer to the group mean will be the better predictor.[38] Individual students take their own individual tests, but the prediction is optimized by relating the observed score to the average of the student's group, where the nature and boundaries of the grouping are entirely at the judgment of the statistician or policymaker. In a place like the United States, where race and ethnicity are central to identity, these are most likely to define the grouping used in statistical procedure and reporting. But many other groupings are equally plausible. For example, in places like Quebec, Belgium, or Peru, language is the much more salient axis of social distinction within those societies, and this is generally how observations are grouped instead.

Groupings are informative to the extent that they have distinct distributions of values. In the muscle mass distributions shown earlier, it is clear that knowing the race group is not informative about the expected value for an individual. Taking non-Hispanic Black and white men, for example, the average lean mass was about 60 kilograms, and 95 percent of values fell within a range of roughly 41 to 78 kilograms. For white men, it was an average of 58 kilograms, and 95 percent of values fell within the range roughly from 42 to 75 kilograms. What makes the race group useless here is that the difference between the averages is tiny (about 2 kilograms) compared to the range within each race group (about 36 kilograms). But there do exist quantities of interest for which race grouping could be informative. For example, we saw earlier that accumulated assets (wealth) in the United States have a much more nonoverlapping distribution between non-Hispanic Blacks and whites. Half of all Black households have assets valued below $20,000, but this is true of only a fifth of white households.[39] Likewise, three out of four Black households have assets less than $100,000, which is true of only about two out of every five white households. If I tell you that a household has $500,000 in assets, you could bet that it is a white household instead of a Black one and be right most of the time.

Therefore, it is important when deciding whether or not to group predictions that we consider whether the proposed grouping is informative. This can be complicated by the fact that the observed differences can also be confounded, as described in chapter 4. In the wealth example, Black populations in the United States tend to live in the poorest states with the lowest wages and property values. For example, the states with the highest proportions of Black citizens are Mississippi (38 percent Black) and Louisiana (33 percent Black). These two are the fiftieth and forty-seventh poorest states in the country, respectively.[40] What this means is that comparing race groups within additional stratifications, like state in this instance, can reveal race to be much less informative than it appears crudely. This presents an ongoing dilemma in debates over the use of race and ethnicity in prediction equations because it can often appear that biological or physiological traits are differentially distributed when in fact this reflects aspects of the social environment. This means that the further stratified contrasts can show race to be irrelevant. A raging debate right now of this sort continues over racial and ethnic differences in birthweight distributions and other measures of perinatal and infant growth.

A child is at high risk of something bad happening during pregnancy, birth, and early life if they are far from the average weight in the population at the same age. In fact, some measures are specifically defined as percentiles. "Small for gestational age," for instance, is a common measure that compares a child's weight to the population average at each week of gestation and defines a child as being small if they are in the lowest 10 percent. But this raises the question of whether a child should be compared to all other children or, more usefully, to children from their same subpopulation. If the latter, this raises the question: Who is their subpopulation? Should it be their country? Their ethnicity? Their race? Their social class stratum? The question of which subpopulation a child belongs to remains a somewhat subjective judgment on the part of the scientist who defines a clinical algorithm.

It is uncontroversial that fetuses and babies should be compared to others of their same sex because everyone agrees that infant girls have better outcomes than boys despite having systematically smaller birthweights by 100 grams or so. This sex difference is taken to be universal and rooted in biology. But many authors have gone even further and asserted that normative values must be defined country by country,[41] and that children of immigrant women should be compared to others from the country of the mother's origin.[42] In 2015, the U.S. National Institute of Child Health and Human Development (NICHD) published new fetal growth standards that were stratified by race and ethnicity, using the standard U.S. census categories.[43] In contrast, other authors have asserted that apparent national, racial, and ethnic differences are just proxies for socioeconomic differences. The international team of investigators who conducted the INTERGROWTH Study asserted that although the average baby is observed to differ in size from place to place or group to group, this need not be the case. They argued that all human babies can potentially be roughly the same size when mothers are healthy and well-nourished in favorable environments.[44] The INTERGROWTH Study was a large international survey in a diverse set of countries but with inclusion criteria that restricted to women experiencing

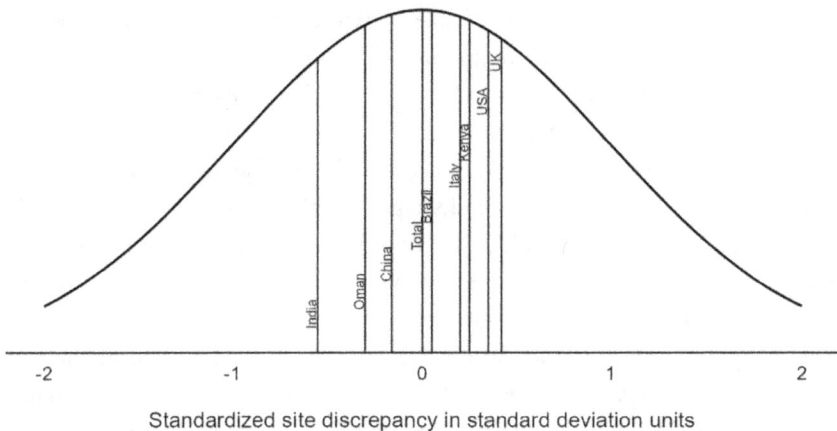

Standardized site discrepancy in standard deviation units

Figure 7.8 Newborn baby head circumference (INTERGROWTH Study).

Source: José Villar et al., "The Likeness of Fetal Growth and Newborn Size Across Non-Isolated Populations in the INTERGROWTH-21st Project: The Fetal Growth Longitudinal Study and Newborn Cross-Sectional Study," *Lancet Diabetes and Endocrinology* 2, no. 10 (2014): 781–92.

pregnancy under "ideal" social and material conditions. When participants were recruited in this way, the investigators observed no important differences in infant size between sites around the world (figure 7.8).

The NICHD investigators remained unpersuaded, however, and doubled down on the necessity for race- and ethnicity-specific fetal growth charts for optimal prediction. However, in 2022, they added a new "unified" category for individuals who do not identify with any one of the standard U.S. census racial and ethnic groups.[45]

Just as ideal infant weights have been racially tailored, so have adult weights. As explained earlier, a standard measure of adiposity is BMI, which is weight (in kilograms) divided by height (in meters) squared. Medical and public health authorities in the United States and in international agencies like the World Health Organization have settled on 30 kg/m^2 as the cut point for defining an adult as obese and 25 kg/m^2 for indicating an adult is overweight, across genders and all adult ages. Nonetheless, many researchers have suggested that these cut points should instead be tailored to the racial and ethnic variations in underlying risks for metabolic diseases, such as type 2 diabetes. Using more than a million patients from the British National Health Service, for example, Rishi Caleyachetty and colleagues determined that to flag the same diabetes risk that a white Briton faces with BMI of 30 kg/m^2, the "obesity" cut point should be set to 23.9 kg/m^2 for South Asians in the United Kingdom and 28.1 kg/m^2 for Black Britons.[46] To label 23.9 kg/m^2 as obese seems a bit of a stretch based on a common-sense definition of the word. For example, Google tells me that the American actor Brad Pitt is 180 centimeters tall and weighs 78 kilograms, giving him a BMI of about 24.1 kg/m^2. That would qualify him as obese if he were South Asian but doesn't even approach overweight status as a white person. To solve this mystery of how apparently slim people could be considered obese, Kapoor and colleagues proposed that South Asians suffer from the phenomenon of *normal weight obesity*.[47] This apparent absurdity arises from using the English word *obesity* to represent risk of metabolic diseases that are affected by a large number of factors beyond body weight, including diet composition, physical activity, and pollution.

Although we might legitimately aim to more aggressively surveil populations who are at greater risk for outcomes, the tailoring of health cut points to racial and ethnic groups rests on questionable premises of generalization across place and time. South Asians around the world do not all share the same social and material environment, and whatever environment they are in now may not be the same as they will find tomorrow. In a classic study conducted in the mid-1970s, epidemiologist Michael Marmot considered the gradient in coronary heart disease risk in Japanese men, which was low in Japan, intermediate in Hawaii, and high in California.[48] Among the immigrants in the United States, he studied degree of acculturation and found that the most traditional group of Japanese Americans had heart disease risk as low as that observed back in Japan, whereas the group that most enthusiastically adopted American ways in their new homeland showed threefold to fivefold higher risk. In short, it was not their race or ethnicity that was most relevant but their diet and behavior. Japanese as a group might have higher or lower risk than some other group, but this observation does not imply that knowing a person is Japanese is the key information for gauging their risk of heart disease.

Finally, in discussing prediction, one must also confront the circularity of past bias feeding back into new predictions. This problem persists because we must always use our knowledge of the world to calibrate our predictions, and so if this knowledge is faulty, then the error is recycled into every new prediction. Consider the longstanding diagnostic advice to physicians in training: "When you hear hoof-beats, look for horses, not zebras." Rare things happen rarely, and common things happen commonly. So if you have to guess, you are better off putting your money on the most common cause.

Now recall the classic 1988 paper by Marti Loring and Brian Powell that was mentioned in chapter 2.[49] The authors constructed an ambiguous psychiatric case presentation and randomly assigned it to be from one of five categories, the four possible combinations of Black or white and male or female and a fifth group without demographic information. These profiles were then assigned a diagnosis by nearly three hundred psychiatrists who returned questionnaires through the mail. Even though the vignettes were identical except for the demographic information, the proportions of the different diagnoses varied substantially by the randomly assigned sex and race of the hypothetical patients. For example, Black men were much more likely to be diagnosed with paranoid schizophrenia, revealing that clinicians perceived these patients as more violent and dangerous than the identical white patients. Furthermore, most of the clinicians who claimed to have insufficient information to form a diagnosis had the vignettes without demographic identifiers. Based on the randomized design, we can clearly attribute the differential diagnosis to bias in the minds of the psychiatrists, but it may be a step too far to label this as racist in the sense of an irrational animus. The reason is that a psychiatrist familiar with the published prevalences of psychiatric conditions in 1988 would have been aware that Black men did supposedly have a higher prevalence of paranoid schizophrenia compared to other groups.[50] The respondents might have therefore simply been trying to implement the wisdom of horses-not-zebras to judge that paranoid schizophrenia was a more likely diagnosis in a group for which it was believed to be more common. This apparent racial difference is then recycled into the next set of statistics to perpetuate the belief.[51]

Economists have long discussed this phenomenon as *statistical discrimination* and have differentiated it from *taste-based discrimination*, which is the kind that arises from simply not liking certain groups of people.[52] It is clearly rational to base one's predictions on knowledge about the world, but three dilemmas arise. The first is that the person may be mistaken about the data that exist, a second is that they may integrate those data poorly into their decision-making, and a third is the circularity described earlier, that the data that exist might themselves be the result of historical biases.[53] This same phenomenon is now discussed widely under the rubric of *algorithmic bias*, especially in the context of artificial intelligence programs that rely on "big data" repositories for context with which to improve assignments and predictions.[54]

Take the example of a recent paper by the economist Renée Adams and colleagues, which considered gender discrimination in the sale prices of paintings at art auctions.[55] Examining almost two million auction transactions in forty-nine countries, they found that paintings by women were priced more than 40 percent lower on average. They then conducted a number of analyses and experiments to try to explain this gap. In one experiment, they generated works of art using artificial intelligence software and then labeled these with recognizably male or female artist names. They found that work attributed to female artists was appraised at lower values than work attributed to male artists. But there are two interpretations to this observed difference. One is that the raters were biased against women artists in an irrational way, what economists would call a *taste-based bias*. But another equally plausible interpretation is that the raters were not biased at all but rather simply aware that female artists in the real world are paid less for their paintings and so they calibrate their own ratings accordingly. Analyses in the paper by Adams and colleagues demonstrated that artistic ability does not differ by gender. For example, study subjects failed to predict the gender of an artist better than chance when shown an anonymized painting. Nonetheless, predicting a lower price for a painting by a woman is the "right" answer in the sense that it may better reflect the prevailing reality in auction data. The idea of statistical discrimination is that study subjects bias their price estimations lower for female artists because they believe that auction bidders do so in the real world and so they use that knowledge to improve their accuracy. This kind of price differential might conceivably disappear if auctions were held with bidders blinded to the artist's name, in the same way that symphony orchestra auditions are conducted behind a screen to prevent discrimination in hiring.[56] Until such a policy change, however, it is impossible to distinguish gender bias in a current appraiser from historical gender bias in the database used by the appraiser to calibrate their new judgments.

In a seemingly objective world of data, we often imagine that categorization and prediction could be done rationally, dispassionately, and fairly. Yet there are limitations to this ideal. Because we tend to rely on our existing notions for what categorizations are most obvious to us and we tend to calibrate our predictions according to the patterns observed in the extant world, we always run the risk of recycling our collective and historical prejudices and stereotypes back into our contemporary prejudices and stereotypes. This is one of the many ways in which science remains a stubbornly *social* process, one subject to our individual and collective human frailties.

CHAPTER VIII

Filters and Screens

A great deal of evidence about racial and ethnic disparities has been published in scientific journals and government reports. Much of this apparent evidence is driven by a somewhat convoluted statistical practice that is nonetheless a ubiquitous expectation in scientific publications across almost all disciplines. This is the *null hypothesis significance test*. It is a simple statistical maneuver that has been used for the last hundred years or so. It may seem obscure to a nonstatistician, but it is behind a great number of the suspicious claims that are asserted in published research. So, with apologies to less quantitative readers, I think it is worth wrestling with the basic details of this fiasco.

Many leading statisticians have decried the mischief wrought by misuse of the null hypothesis significance text, and yet its grip on scientific publishing remains firm. In 2016 the American Statistical Association (ASA) published an assessment calling for abandoning null hypothesis significance tests as the standard of scientific evidence in journal publications.[1] Even the U.S. Supreme Court reached a similar conclusion in 2011 when it ruled against a pharmaceutical company that did not disclose adverse events because the data had not been subjected to such tests.[2] These and similar pleas have mostly been ignored. Old habits die hard, even when they are the source of so much confusion and error. In fact, the ASA statement begins with the obvious question of why a malignant practice would remain so pervasive: Why do we continue to teach this approach to our students in university statistics classes? The answer offered is that it's necessary to prepare students for the prevailing expectations of journal editors and grant reviewers, even if those expectations are misguided. And why do journal editors and grant reviewers continue to have such misguided expectations? Because this is what they were taught in their university statistics classes. And so we have a portrait of a classic self-reinforcing social pathology.[3]

Significance testing begins by invoking a null hypothesis, which is meant to be a statement of the existing state of knowledge or the result that is not supposed to surprise anyone—the default belief. Then in contrast to this null hypothesis, there must be an alternate hypothesis, which can be as general as "something other than the null" or more specific. For example, if the null hypothesis is that a new drug is no different from a placebo, the alternative hypothesis can be simply that they are different but is usually more specifically that the new drug is better. Many racial and ethnic disparities are studied in this way, where the null hypothesis is generally that groups have the same prevalence of some condition or that a treatment works the same way in every group.

Statisticians use the data gathered to assess whether the observations are consistent with the stated null hypothesis. If there is enough evidence in the data to conclude that the estimated difference would not likely be observed if the null were true, then it can be logically asserted that the null must be false. One is then left with no logical choice other than to embrace the alternative. The decision is often expressed by calculating a *p-value*, which is a hypothetical statistical score representing the likelihood of observing the study data if the null hypothesis were true. More precisely, the *p*-value is the probability of observing the estimated parameter or a more extreme value if the null hypothesis were true. Readers of scientific research will see these *p*-values scattered liberally throughout the published papers, especially in tables of results. This score is then often compared to a rejection criterion to facilitate a binary decision. The cut point is most commonly set by social convention, such that one will make a false rejection of the null only 5 percent of the time.

For a concrete example of calculating *p*-values, statisticians are fond of coin flipping because the outcome of the flip is close to random and the binary outcome means that the probabilities are easy to calculate.[4] In this case, my null hypothesis is that the coin is fair. If I flip the coin several times and exactly half the flips are "heads," then I have no evidence against this null hypothesis. But suppose I flip the coin three times and get three heads. My alternative hypothesis is simply "this is not a fair coin," by which I mean that the probability of obtaining heads is not exactly half. Recall that the p-value is the probability of the observed data or some result even more extreme, assuming that the null hypothesis is true. In this case, there is nothing more extreme, so it would be just the probability of getting three heads in a row on a fair coin, which is $0.5 \times 0.5 \times 0.5 = 0.125$. Likewise, the p-value for four heads in a row would be 0.0625. Because the prevailing social convention mentioned earlier for declaring a result to be "significant" is $p < 0.05$, these four consecutive heads would still not be enough for us to reject the hypothesis of a fair coin. But the fifth consecutive head leads to a p-value of 0.03, and with that result, we cross this threshold and so are supposed to stop believing in the fair coin because such a result, occurring by chance only three times per one hundred times, seems too improbable.

The flaws in this approach and the opportunities for misuse and abuse are almost limitless. For example, the null may be a strawman hypothesis that nobody would believe, like the absence of a racial disparity in police stops. Moreover, in large datasets, it becomes impossible to find any two groups perfectly equal in anything, meaning that the null can always be rejected if the sample size is large enough. Scientists may obtain a p-value that rejects the null hypothesis as unlikely, but their obtained estimate can be even more unlikely.[5] Take the earlier coin-flipping example; we rejected the null hypothesis of a fair coin because the data would only occur three out of a hundred times. But how many unfair coins have you actually come across in your life? Probably far fewer than three per one hundred. Small datasets often lead to accepting the null even when it is false, and large datasets lead to rejecting the null when it is qualitatively true. Scientists who want to reject the null hypothesis can conduct many tests until they get lucky, and scientists who don't want to reject the null can make enough adjustments to prevent themselves from doing so. So, all in all, this method allows for insincere investigators to demonstrate whatever it is they wish to show, and even sincere investigators often make errors in the technique or interpretation that jeopardize the validity of the work. One enormously frequent error, for example, is to make a statistical test of a treatment in one racial group, say whites, and make a separate test in another racial group, say Blacks. If one rejects the null for one group and not for the other, many investigators are tempted to conclude that the treatment works for only one race and not for the other. This is erroneous because it is not the hypothesis being tested. The conclusion that one race is different from the other would legitimately arise instead from a single test of the null hypothesis that the treatment response is equivalent versus the alternative that it is different. This error is endemic in published papers and often missed by peer reviewers and editors.[6]

Let me give a concrete example to show what this looks like in practice. I hesitate to single out any one paper because this is such a common error, but it's important to keep on guard for the kind of language that signals this erroneous statistical interpretation. Here is one rather typical instance of this phenomenon. A group of researchers from San Francisco was interested in the effects of the so-called Mediterranean diet on cognitive aging, so they conducted an elaborate study and published their findings in the prestigious *Journals of Gerontology Series A* in 2014.[7] The authors followed more than two thousand adults in their seventies for about a decade. A little less than 40 percent of the subjects were Black. Using questionnaires on frequently consumed foods, they classified the participants in relation to their adherence to a Mediterranean diet, which is low in meat and high in olive oil. They also gave the participants periodic mental acuity assessments and calculated global cognitive scores that ranged from 0 to 100. They compared trajectories of decline in these scores by diet and race. The authors summarized their results this way: "We found a significant correlation between strong adherence to the Mediterranean diet and a slower rate of cognitive decline among African American, but not white, older adults. Our study is the first to show a possible race-specific association between the Mediterranean diet and cognitive decline."[8]

Of course, the Black and white participants in this study might differ in many ways that could affect cognitive decline, such as degree of schooling or income, so you might already be thinking of confounding as discussed in chapter 4. To address this concern, the authors used a regression model to hold constant other measured characteristics of the participants. They included in this model their available indicators of age, sex, educational attainment, body mass index, whether they were current smokers, reported physical activity, depression, diabetes, total energy intake, and socioeconomic status. If we accept the statistical assumptions of this model and the self-reports of these characteristics, we can assume that the results are not confounded by these factors. Of course, they can still be confounded by other things, like air pollution, and this is mentioned in the discussion as a study limitation. One curious aspect of this adjustment is the inclusion of total calories because it implies that any effect of the Mediterranean diet cannot be through reducing calories. Rather, if a person adheres to this diet by eating less meat, they are assumed by this adjustment to compensate by eating more of something else to replace those missing calories.

Although these other aspects are interesting and relevant, let's focus on the use of significance testing to drive the interpretation of the paper. Recall that a significance test involves a null hypothesis that may be rejected if the data are found to be incompatible. In this case, the authors' null hypothesis is that cognitive decline is the same in people with high and low diet scores, where a high diet score reflects the Mediterranean pattern of foods, after adjustment for the measured covariates listed earlier. If we reject this null, we accept instead that diet score and cognitive decline are associated, and if we can rule out noncausal explanations for this association, like confounding or selection bias, then we might start advising people to eat more like Greeks and Spaniards. The authors estimate an adjusted effect, which is the average change in cognitive score over the follow-up period in those with high diet scores minus the change in those with low diet scores. Everyone declines over time, sadly, but the authors are concerned with whether the lower diet score group declines faster, and they fit these regression models separately for Blacks and for whites. With each modeled estimate of effect comes a p-value, which is interpreted as the probability of observing an estimate that large or larger if the null hypothesis were true. In this case, the null hypothesis being true means that the Mediterranean diet has no effect on cognitive decline. Therefore, a small p-value leads to rejection of the null hypothesis and thus would support an association between the diet and the cognition measures. The reported effect estimates were 0.09 points for whites and 0.22 points for Blacks. Remember that the cognitive score ranges from 0 to 100, so a contrast of 0.09 points between diet groups over the follow-up represents less than one thousandth of the range. The p-value for whites was 0.14 and the p-value for Blacks was 0.01 (figure 8.1). Recall that the somewhat arbitrary convention is to tolerate a false rejection one out of twenty times, which corresponds to a p-value cut point of 0.05 as the threshold for declaring an estimate to be *statistically significant*. Therefore, by conventional practice, the null is rejected for Blacks but not for whites, and this is why the authors have declared that olive oil is only good for the cognition of Black people.

Sadly, this is all completely normative nutritional epidemiology, and the statistical approach here would be equally embraced across most of biomedicine and social science. This is why the peer reviewers of this article checked off on these methods and it was published in a top journal. But

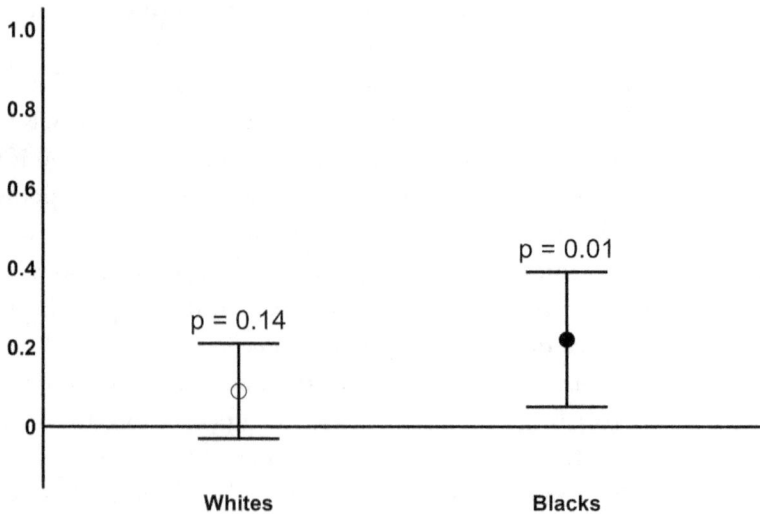

Figure 8.1 Association between diet score and cognition trajectories.

Source: Alain Koyama et al., "Association Between the Mediterranean Diet and Cognitive Decline in a Bira-cial Population," *Journals of Gerontology Series A: Biomedical Sciences and Medical Sciences* 70, no. 3 (2015): 354–59.

look more closely and you'll see the problem. Consider each estimate, 0.09 for whites and 0.22 for Blacks, as a new null hypothesis, and construct the range of values around each estimate that would be judged to not be "significantly" different at the same $p = 0.05$ criterion. This range therefore represents all the effect magnitudes that are roughly consistent with the observed data for each group, called the *95 percent confidence interval.* This interval is reported by the authors in their paper as −0.03 to 0.21 for whites and 0.05 to 0.39 for Blacks. The interval is wider for Blacks, of course, because they are less than 40 percent of the sample; the interval is 0.24 units wide for whites and 0.34 units wide for Blacks. Smaller samples sizes generate more uncertainty about the location of the estimates because they vary more from one iteration of the study to the next. Think of it this way. If I flip a fair coin four times, my observed proportion of heads can easily be anything from 0 to 100 percent. But if I flip the same coin a million times, I am guaranteed to see something much closer to 50 percent heads. In the same way, the sample of whites has less uncertainty about the location of its estimate just because there are more observations in the dataset. Size matters! One can visualize this by plotting the adjusted estimates and their

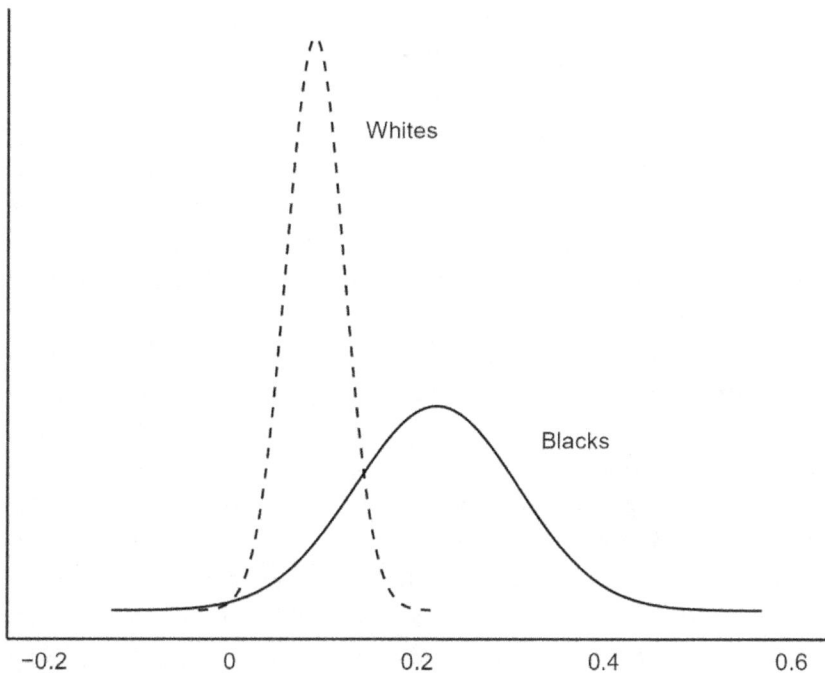

Figure 8.2 Schematic representation of adjusted effect estimates and their sampling distributions based on the reported 95% confidence intervals, by race.

Source: Alain Koyama et al., "Association Between the Mediterranean Diet and Cognitive Decline in a Biracial Population," *Journals of Gerontology Series A: Biomedical Sciences and Medical Sciences* 70, no. 3 (2015): 354–59.

sampling distributions based on the information in the confidence intervals that was reported by the authors (figure 8.2).[9]

The white estimate is centered around 0.09 and the Black estimate around 0.22, and each has an uncertainty associated with sampling error, which is the luck of drawing people from the population with different diets and cognitive fates. Remember that the range of values shown is the range of estimates that would not generate a $p < 0.05$ when tested against the observed effect. The thing to notice here is that almost all white values are entirely consistent with the Black data. The white estimate of 0.09 is inside the Black 95 percent confidence interval and therefore not statistically distinct. In fact, the authors tested each race group separately, with a null hypothesis of 0 for the effect of diet on cognitive change, and the white estimate yielded a p-value of 0.14, higher than 0.05, and so was considered "not significant." But if the white estimate were to be instead tested against the Black estimate, the *p*-value in that case is even larger (*p* = 0.22) and therefore even further from the significance threshold.[10] The authors concluded that Blacks and whites were fundamentally different in their response to this diet, boasting in the press release that their paper was the first to show a "race-specific association between the Mediterranean diet and cognitive decline." In fact, there is little evidence here that Black and white effects were dissimilar, as is immediately obvious from the overlapping likelihoods plotted in figure 8.2.

Again, there is nothing special about the methods in this paper. This happens all the time. The same error is committed when considering differences by sex or any other characteristic, but the problem is exacerbated by differences in sample sizes between the groups, and racial/ethnic minorities tend to have smaller representation in studies exactly because they are minorities. Sometimes authors contradict themselves, pointing out this erroneous difference while also disproving it elsewhere in the same paper. For example, a SNP (pronounced "snip") is a single nucleotide polymorphism, meaning a base pair substitution at one DNA location on the genome. Pieter Stijnen and colleagues investigated the association between various SNPs and obesity and reported in a synthesis of studies that three SNPs in the PCSK1 gene were significantly associated with obesity, but not in everyone.[11] Rather, they concluded that there was an association with obesity in the Caucasian population but not among Hispanics.

The effect estimate of interest in this case was an *odds ratio*, abbreviated OR. An OR here is the probability of being obese divided by the probability of not being obese (i.e., the odds of obesity) in one group; this number is then divided by the comparable odds in another group. Thus, an OR, which is a very frequent effect parameter in epidemiological studies, is a ratio of two ratios and so involves three separate divisions. You might think that this is a strange effect parameter to use and you'd be right, but its popularity follows from some very convenient mathematical properties, especially in designs called *case-control studies*, which dominate the study of genetic effects. I'll have more to say about odds ratios in chapter 9.

The association for Caucasians reported by the authors was an OR of 1.17, with a 95 percent confidence interval of 1.09 to 1.27. For the much smaller number of Hispanics in the dataset, it was an OR of 1.50, with a 95 percent confidence interval of 0.65 to 3.48. Plotting these as likelihoods again drives home the fact that the Hispanic estimate is highly imprecise and that

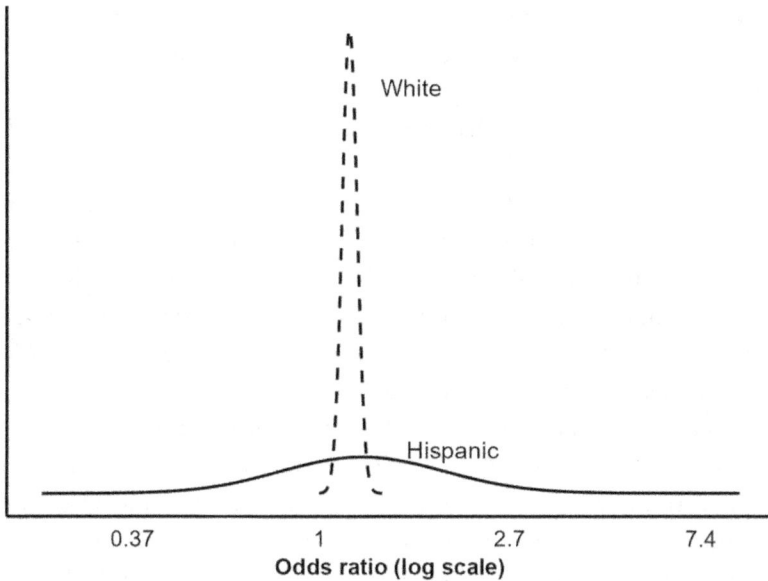

Figure 8.3 Schematic representation of summary odds ratios (log scale) and their sampling distributions based on the reported 95% confidence intervals, for whites and Hispanics.

Source: Pieter Stijnen et al., "The Association of Common Variants in PCSK1 with Obesity: A HuGE Review and Meta-Analysis," *American Journal of Epidemiology* 180, no. 11 (2014): 1051–65.

it was in no way incompatible with the Caucasian estimate (figure 8.3). The authors themselves noted this in the published paper, at one point conducting a significance test specifically positing a null hypothesis of ethnic homogeneity and obtaining a large p-value of 0.43 and therefore noting correctly that ethnic groups did *not* differ significantly. And yet somehow this point was lost by the time they reached the conclusion, where they stated that they had established a significant contribution of the three PCSK1 SNPs to the genetic predisposition for obesity in an "ethnicity-dependent fashion." Subsequent modeling has shown that many similar claims of ethnic-specific genetic effects that appear in the literature are likely to arise from these sorts of underpowered comparisons.[12]

Another common problem with significance testing is the multiplicity problem, by which multiple testing distorts the interpretation of a test. Consider that a small p-value means that the observed effect or an even more extreme effect would not be expected if the null were true. We reject the null in this circumstance simply because we believe that rare things should not happen very often because they are rare. But low-probability events can happen easily if you allow enough tries. For example, the probability of drawing a straight in a five-card poker hand, meaning any five cards in numerical order, is less than half a percent. It happens a little bit less than once in every 250 deals. That's pretty rare. But if you deal me a hundred hands, I have about a one-third chance of encountering a straight, and that doesn't seem so rare at all anymore.[13] The same applies to testing and rejecting the null hypothesis, which means that in any complex analysis, we can test enough things so that something will come out as "significant" eventually, just by dumb luck. In the trade, this is generally referred to as *fishing*. Social and biomedical scientists love to go fishing.

Multiple racial and ethnic groups provide many opportunities to get lucky, in the sense of detecting an apparent association even when the null hypothesis is true, meaning there really isn't a correlation. This is how some clever researchers managed to discover in 2006 that Canadians born under the astrological sign Leo had a higher probability of gastrointestinal hemorrhage ($p = 0.04$), whereas Sagittarians had a higher probability of a humerus fracture ($p = 0.01$).[14] The authors considered any astrological difference for any of more than two hundred medical conditions among 10.6 million residents of Ontario. Such a high sample size and so many possible conditions guaranteed that some connections would be "significant" by chance. The urge to capitalize on chance in this way is especially acute when there's a lot of money at stake, as in the case of a potential pharmaceutical treatment, for which a great deal is invested in early development and the difference between financial success and ruin relies on the results of a randomized trial. If the overall effect is not significant, it can be very tempting to rifle through subgroups, including racial and ethnic categories, hunting for some significant effect somewhere.

One such example was the case of AIDSVAX, a potential human immunodeficiency virus (HIV) vaccine that was developed by the pharmaceutical company Genentech and that, in 2003, failed to show a positive effect at the end of a three-year study of more than five thousand volunteers spread across roughly forty clinical sites.[15] Desperate to avoid an abject failure after this substantial investment, the company quickly pivoted to intriguing evidence that the vaccine might have a positive response only in the small number of Black and Asian study subjects. At the end of the trial, HIV was contracted by 5.7 percent of the vaccinated and 5.8 percent of the placebo group, yielding the overall null result. And yet among the Black volunteers, the company excitedly reported 76 percent fewer HIV infections among the vaccinated, corresponding to a p-value of less than 0.02 and therefore below the magic significance threshold of 0.05.

But it did not take long for this attempted deflection to fall apart. Only 314 of the study participants were Black. In this small group, 111 were assigned the placebo, and nine of them (8.1 percent) became HIV positive. Among the 203 who received the active vaccine, four contracted HIV (2 percent). This contrast generated the apparently large proportional effect but based on a mere handful of cases.[16] Predictably, these apparent effects did not hold up. A subsequent trial failed to show any effect of the vaccine, and it was quickly abandoned. Although a few researchers publicly speculated about some special genetic traits among Blacks that might relate to HIV infection, most scientists shamed the company for this desperate statistical impropriety.[17] "We've seen this in AIDS trials before, when the results are not acceptable for the investigators. They go fishing for some answer they like better," wrote the epidemiologist Gregg Gonsalves.[18] A small p-value is supposed to rule out a chance finding, but if investigators troll through dozens or hundreds of subgroups, that's exactly what they will get.

Another aspect of significance testing to worry about is the supposed error rate. Rejecting the null hypothesis at $p < 0.05$ means that about 5 percent of the time researchers will reject the null hypothesis when it is actually true. This promised frequency of errors will only hold if there are no other sources of bias, like confounding, selection bias, or measurement error. In the context of an ideal randomized trial in which there is no dropout, no measurement error, and so on, then with a large sample size, we can indeed be confident that the 5 percent theoretical error rate will hold. Many observational studies also rely on significance testing, however, and rarely would we ever believe that these studies have no confounding or other biases.[19] When you consider the comparison of study subjects by race or ethnicity, these factors are very far from randomly assigned, which implies that they are in fact correlated with a great many things. In this setting, we would expect a significance test for any one selected factor to have an error rate very far from the theoretical standard. This is because no matter what is adjusted for as a confounder, something else is sure to be imbalanced between the groups.

Say you read a study asserting some biological difference between Black men and white men that explains the observed excess of prostate cancer incidence or mortality in Black men. The authors will generally conduct a significance test for the role of some tumor characteristic to identify it as the explanation for the disparity. Recognizing that Black and white men might differ by socioeconomic status, which has implications for diet, occupation, pollution, and other relevant environmental factors, they would generally seek a marker of social status for which they would adjust the results. This might be, for instance, how many years of attained education a subject has. But even at the same educational level, two men of different races would be expected to differ in income. Even if some more meticulous authors adjusted for education *and* income together, two men with the same education and income but different races would be expected to differ in financial assets. You can see that one can go on like this forever, finding further disparities within any set of factors that are set to be mathematically equal. In a racially stratified society, one can expect that the residual inequality in unmeasured factors will always persist, no matter what is added to the model as an adjustment. Seen in this way, the model can never hope to provide enough covariate balance to interpret the significance test as a statement about the factor of interest, rather than being about the unmeasured variables that remain out of the model. Add to this the commonly crude categorization of the measured adjustment variables, as well as missing data, and the problem looks hopeless for significance testing in this setting.[20]

This is not merely a hypothetical example. It applies more or less to most of the published biomedical literature on topics such as racial disparities in prostate cancer. Consider one highly cited paper on the topic. The pathologist Francesca Khani and colleagues examined tumor nodules extracted from 105 Black and 113 white prostate cancer patients and examined a number of biological and genetic traits.[21] The authors adjusted these racial comparisons only for age, body mass index, and measures of the tumor stage and aggressiveness. They reported small p-values, thus rejecting the null hypothesis, which was that Black and white men with prostate cancer had similar cancer etiologies. Notice that no social factors were considered at all, nor is there any explanation for how representative these particular men might be of any population. The authors only mention that the study subjects were consecutive cases at the same academic medical center and that because this hospital only accepted patients who had insurance, they must at least have been equal in that single social dimension.

This prostate cancer disparity paper concluded, like so many others, that the significant contrast between Black and white men in genetic characteristics of the prostate cancer tumors signals a racially distinct etiology that might be relevant for differential diagnostics and treatment. Not only has this particular paper been highly cited, but the result was even patented by the authors.[22] It is just one of thousands upon thousands of published papers that take a similar statistical approach, treating people as randomly assigned to their racial and ethnic groups, conditional on a just a few measured factors like age and body mass index, and then using the rejection of the statistical null as "proof" of essential differences even while myriad social and environmental differences are ignored. The null hypothesis significance test is designed to rule out an alternate explanation that observed differences arise simply from the luck of having drawn an imbalanced sample, but in this setting in which one is studying racial and ethnic disparities, the null hypothesis has no real prima facie credibility. Remember that a randomized trial guarantees by design that the treatment is the only factor that differs between the two groups. In a study of prostate cancer risk factors between Black and white men, given how profoundly racial identity shapes every aspect of life in the United States, it makes much more sense to start out instead with the null hypothesis that everything in the social environment will be different between these groups.[23]

In the same way that a null hypothesis significance test for the difference between racial or ethnic groups is structurally and intractably confounded, as explained earlier, a significance test of some other factor in an ethnically mixed population can be just as hopeless because of these same ubiquitous differences. In genetic epidemiology, this is recognized under the term *population stratification*.[24] A common technique in genetic epidemiology is to go down the whole genome, testing SNPs one after another to see whether the variants are differentially more or less common among cases of a disease than among noncases. In a seminal article from 1994, the geneticist Eric Lander warned that this strategy could fail in an ethnically diverse dataset. "In a mixed population, any trait present at a higher frequency in an ethnic group will show positive association with any allele that also happens to be more common in that group," Lander wrote.[25] To demonstrate this, he offered the example that a naïve geneticist might attempt a study among the San Francisco population to find the genetic variation that determines an ability to eat with chopsticks. There are many highly variable segments of human DNA, and Lander gives the example of the human leukocyte antigen (HLA) system, a set of genes on chromosome 6 that encode cell-surface proteins for regulating the immune system. There are many, many different alleles at these loci, and therefore, different populations inevitably show different patterns. Any allele that is more or less common among Asians than among whites will reject the hypothesis of no association. That's because, as far as the researcher is concerned, this difference is not due to chance, and therefore, this variant will be "discovered" as a determinant of chopstick use. The conventional solution to this problem has long been to stratify on ethnicity in all genetic analyses so that populations under study are presumably more homogeneous.

Lander's example is fanciful, but population stratification has led to real blunders in genetic epidemiology due to unrecognized ethnic heterogeneity and an uncritical allegiance to null hypothesis significance testing. One famous example comes from a study of the same HLA system and its association with diabetes among the Pima, an Indigenous ethnicity in Arizona.[26] The authors "discovered" the connection between the HLA region and diabetes, but it turned out to be confounded by European admixture in the Pima because the Pima with more white ancestry also had different social status and diet and, therefore, a different prevalence of diabetes. This is just garden-variety confounding, as discussed in chapter 4, but the important point here is that null hypothesis significance tests are premised on there being no confounding. Instead, they assume the kind of pure experimental conditions that prevail in a randomized trial, so that all other potential causes of the outcome would be balanced between the two treatment groups. In the case of searching for a genetic cause of diabetes, the nongenetic causes (social position, diet, physical activity, and so on) are necessarily tied to race and ethnicity in a racially stratified society. In the case of the Pima, those individuals with the most purely Indigenous ancestry were found differentially in the least socially privileged positions. This kind of confounding has sometimes been referred to as "structural" because it arises from an overarching social structure that assigns risk factors based on racialized power relations, not from a coin flip, as would happen in a trial.[27]

Null hypothesis significance tests function as a kind of a filter, qualifying some results for publication and not others, but they do a terrible job in this role. For example, one consequence of setting up a p-value threshold of 5 percent for publication is the "regression to the mean" problem described in chapter 7. Because the most extreme estimates pass the threshold, they tend to end up being smaller in magnitude when replicated, meaning that "significant" findings are overestimates of the true effect sizes.[28] One could go on and on with more complaints about this procedure, and indeed, there are entire books devoted to the damage done by this kind of statistical testing.[29] But this chapter is focused on the particular problems associated with testing in relation to racial or ethnic disparities, and one can easily draw parallels with the other issues discussed already, like confounding.

Much of the statistical machinery for biomedicine and social science, including statistical testing, arose from experimental settings in which treatments were allocated randomly. All mathematical justifications for the null hypothesis significance procedure are derived under these conditions, and the generalization to observed treatments rather than assigned treatments has always been a bit shaky.[30] Ultimately, the *p*-value is a kind of model, as discussed in chapter 2, and in many applications, it is so far from its original premises that it is simply a very bad model. At some point, we have to be able to recognize the settings in which it can be unhelpful and even harmful. There are places where it will make more or less sense, depending on the specific hypotheses being entertained,[31] but I would aver that, overall, considering the broad swath of published biomedical and social science work, significance testing has done much more harm than good.

In fact, the focus of significance testing is entirely on random errors, the kind that arise because you happened by dumb luck to recruit one person from the population into your study instead of some other person. Random errors are the kind that go away if you simply repeat the study, a way of shuffling the deck. I would argue that for work on race and ethnicity, in most settings, and especially in the era of "big data," random error is the *least* of our problems. The kinds of errors described in the preceding chapters, like confounding, selection bias, and misclassification, are not random errors—they are systematic. For example, if the Pima study that falsely linked the HLA haplotype to diabetes had been done again with fifty thousand participants instead of five thousand, the problem would not go away. In this way, statistical testing has been a red herring, leading us down the garden path, far from where we really want to go.

CHAPTER IX

―――――

Scales, Values, and Preferences

A disparity is just the observation that one measured value is different from another measured value. Holland, for example, has the world's largest average adult height, and there is a disparity in the average heights of Dutch men and women because the male average is 72.4 inches and the female average is 66.9 inches.[1] But how does one quantify this gender disparity? Is it larger or smaller than the gender disparity somewhere else? If we want to compare Holland to another country, say Bolivia, we need to contrast these two average heights mathematically to make a single quantitative summary. The two most common ways to do this are to take the difference (72.4 inches − 66.9 inches = 5.5 inches) or the ratio (72.4 inches/66.9 inches = 1.082). So we could say that Dutch men are 5.5 inches taller than Dutch women or that they are 8.2 percent taller. Both are true statements. It is just that one is an absolute contrast and the other a relative contrast. At first, it might seem that there is no obvious advantage of one scale of contrast over the other. In Bolivia, the height averages for men and women are 66.1 inches and 61.0 inches, for a difference of 5.1 inches or a ratio disparity of 8.4 percent. So in which country is the gender disparity greater? Based on the difference, the disparity is greater in Holland (5.5 > 5.1), but based on the ratio, it is greater in Bolivia (1.082 < 1.084). Each is a legitimate mathematical contrast, and yet they lead to opposite conclusions about where the disparity is greatest. This allows researchers to pick either country as the more disparate and allows them to provide valid quantitative evidence to support their claim either way.

This is very simple math, and yet it is remarkable how much confusion arises over this issue of differences versus ratios for disparity comparisons. The confusion is exacerbated by the overwhelming habit of favoring the ratio contrasts in all government and academic surveillance of disparities. It is not quite clear how this came to be the dominant practice, but almost all disparity statistics are reported in this way. Both scales are mathematically legitimate, of course, but the ratio presentation hides some important information. If one group is twice as likely to get an outcome, that is presented as a ratio of 2.0. But this ratio value could arise from 80 percent versus 40 percent, or 1 percent versus 0.5 percent, or 0.0004 percent versus 0.0002 percent, and so on. This makes it possible for some very small differences to look very large. Say there are two groups being compared for disease risk and the values are 0.0273 percent and 0.0109 percent. The difference is 0.0164 percent, or one extra case per six thousand people, which seems not especially alarming. But this disparity will most often instead be published simply as the ratio 2.50 and interpreted as one group having 150 percent greater risk than the other group,[2] which sounds huge.[3]

There are various arguments about which scale might be more meaningfully interpreted, and that mostly depends on the specific application. Disparities in academic test scores might be more natural on the relative scale because the units are arbitrary and it only matters how one scores in relation to others. For concrete outcomes like death, disease, arrest, or incarceration, however, people experience or don't experience the events individually, not in relation to others. That is, you want your risk of death to be low in *absolute* terms, not merely relative to other people, because you have exactly one life to lose or not lose. Is it reassuring that your airplane has a 10 percent chance of crashing if you're told that this is only half the risk of someone else's airplane?

Think of it this way. Suppose you regularly set aside $10 to go to a favorite pub where the nuts are $1, the beer is $2, and the hamburger is $4. One day you come in and the prices have all changed to $1.50, $3, and $6. "Hey, what's going on?" you ask the bartender. He looks puzzled and replies, "Nothing has changed here. Beer was twice the price of nuts, and it still is, and hamburgers were twice the price of beer, and they still are. Everything is the same." As you stand there with your same $10 bill, you will feel aggrieved by this sudden change because your resources are fixed on the absolute scale and constancy of the relative relations between the prices is not helpful to you. When it comes to your single life or your $10 at the pub, you care about the absolute risk and prices not the relative ones.

It is surprising, therefore, that relative disparities are most often front and center, even when they defy this logic. Take for example a report by the geographer Ian Gregory in the *British Medical Journal*.[4] Gregory was interested in how the disparities in mortality rates between rich and poor districts in Britain and Wales have changed over the twentieth century, and so he examined census and mortality data for the entire population in 1900 and in 2001. There were dramatic improvements in life expectancy over this period. The infant mortality rate fell from 127.6 to 5.4 deaths per one thousand births. Life expectancy for men rose from forty-six to seventy-seven, an additional thirty-one years of life on average. Nonetheless, the most economically deprived districts had about 40 percent higher mortality in 2001, almost the exact same relative excess as observed in 1900. This led to the main conclusion of the article, which is that economic disparities had not budged at all. "The relation between the extremes of deprivation and mortality is as strong today as it was a century ago," concluded the author. A rising tide had lifted all boats on the absolute scale, but because it had lifted them proportionally, the author concluded that no progress had been made whatsoever.

To see how this scale confusion plays out with racial and ethnic disparities, consider the 2010 study in the *American Journal of Public Health* by the epidemiologist Jennifer Orsi and colleagues.[5] The authors were interested in whether health indicator disparities between non-Hispanic Black and non-Hispanic white people widened, narrowed, or stayed the same between 1990 and 2005. They reported that the disparities had worsened for six of fifteen studied outcomes at the national level and eleven of fifteen in Chicago. To understand the calculations in detail, let's drill down into the numerical comparisons for just one of these examined conditions: tuberculosis.

The tuberculosis incidence rate for Black Americans in 1990 was 33.0 cases per 100,000 persons per year, whereas for white Americans, it was 4.2 cases per 100,000 persons per year. The authors reasoned that $33.0 - 4.2$ was a difference of 28.8 excess cases per 100,000 persons per year, where "excess cases" are cases that occur in Black people because they do not share the lower rate experienced by white people. The authors did not present this disparity as $33.0 - 4.2 = 28.8$, however, but instead followed

	Black rate	White rate	Relative disparity
1990	33.0	4.2	(33.0 – 4.2) / 4.2 = 685.7
2005	11.6	1.3	(11.6 – 1.3) / 1.3 = 792.3

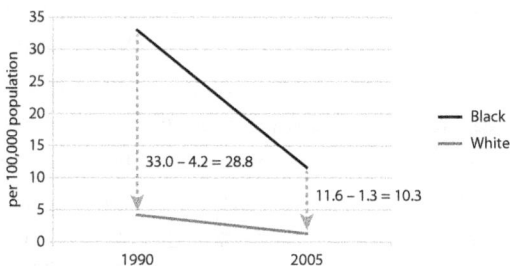

Figure 9.1 Tuberculosis case rate per 100,000 population per year by race.

Source: Jennifer M. Orsi, Helen Margellos-Anast, and Steven Whitman, "Black–White Health Disparities in the United States and Chicago: A 15-Year Progress Analysis," *American Journal of Public Health* 100, no. 2 (2010): 349–56.

the usual convention of reporting this excess *relative* to the white rate and, therefore, described it in their paper as a (28.8/4.2) × 100 percent = 685.7 percent excess.

Fortunately, by 2005, the tuberculosis rate in the United States had plummeted across the board. The authors found that the Black rate was down from 33.0 to 11.6 cases per 100,000 persons per year and that the white rate had fallen from 4.2 to 1.3 cases per 100,000 persons per year. In 2005, this was thus a racial difference of 11.6 − 1.3 = 10.3. This is almost a third of the absolute difference that existed in 1990. But again, the authors reported this excess *relative* to the white rate of 1.3 and therefore described it as a (10.3/1.3) × 100 percent = 792.3 percent excess. By comparing the approximately 700 percent excess rate in 1990 to the approximately 800 percent excess rate in 2005, the authors concluded that racial disparities had *worsened* (figure 9.1). The math is correct, but the conclusion that everything was worse in 2005 seems completely bananas because both groups have improved dramatically.

Look at it this way: in 1990, the difference between the two racial group rates was 33.0 − 4.2 = 28.8 excess cases per 100,000 people per year. That was 28.8 out of every 100,000 Black people who had tuberculosis that year only because their rate was higher than the white rate. By 2005, that excess rate decreased to 11.6 − 1.3 = 10.3 out of every 100,000 Black people who had tuberculosis that year because their rate was higher than the white rate. Thus, the annual number of excess cases for each 100,000 people actually fell to less than half, from 28.8 down to 10.3. This implies many fewer Black people each year had tuberculosis because they were subject to the Black rate instead of the white rate. Surely this should count as progress, but because of the authors' choice of scale, the disparity appeared worse over time even though, in absolute numbers, tuberculosis was much less common in both groups. Some arbitrariness in accounting is unavoidable, in the sense that one must pick a scale and both are mathematically valid. The relative scale necessitates additional arbitrary decisions, like the choice of the denominator. These authors divided by the white rate, but one could have just as legitimately divided by the Black rate. In principle, one could present results on both scales, allowing readers to see both seemingly contradictory truths—that the relative disparity is getting worse while the absolute disparity is getting better. But journal articles have page limits that require parsimony, and presenting both scales might confuse people even more.

I would still argue that the absolute excess risk is the measure that comes closer to capturing the individual harm that motivates a concern over disparities in the first place. After all, groups don't experience disease and death; individuals do. Having 28.8 extra people out of every 100,000 catch tuberculosis is a terrible thing for those individuals. If that number falls to only 10.3 extra people, that means more happy people without tuberculosis, which ought to be considered good news, not bad news. To prefer instead the relative measure interpretation that the latter gap is worse, one is implicitly endorsing the ethical viewpoint that it is the inequality itself that is the inherently bad thing, not the experience of tuberculosis for the individual.[6] This philosophical position is even advanced by some authors, arguing that if the worse-off group is not improving at a *faster* rate than the better-off group, then the disparity is not moving toward equality.[7] But this line of thinking leads to some uncomfortable places. For example, the rate of opioid overdose mortality in the United States has long been higher for whites than for Blacks. Tragically, rates are *increasing* for both groups but more rapidly among Black Americans. Over the last decade or so, the *relative* gap between these two racial groups has been *decreasing*.[8] According to the logic of gauging trends by comparing ratios instead of differences, this would count as an improvement, a movement toward racial equality and away from racial disparity in outcomes—even though more people in both groups are dying every year.

I stated earlier that ratio measures hide some information in descriptive contexts like the example above, but when assessing the effect of a treatment instead of merely monitoring a disparity, the ratio does even worse. Let's suppose we wanted to get the causal effect of ethnicity on a judgment, as we did in the audit studies described in chapter 2. Let's conjure up a hypothetical experiment with fictional data to better explain this point. Say we are interested in a judge's decision to impose pretrial detention on a person charged with a crime. So we conduct a randomized trial in which we present written files describing equivalent defendants to a judge, with all characteristics held constant except for names, switching between names that most people would recognize as Hispanic or Anglo. In this way, we might detect ethnic discrimination in the judge's decision. Of course, the cases brought before the judge involve a wide range of criminal offenses and the defendants have a wide range of background characteristics, like previous arrests. All of these other factors will certainly affect the judge's decision to order preventive detention or not, but we are interested in finding if there are instances in which, holding the large set of background factors constant, the judge's decision would differ depending on the apparent ethnicity of the defendant alone.

Taking the whole population of cases, there are logically only three possible latent types of defendants:

Type A would be ordered held until trial regardless of their apparent ethnicity.

Type B would be released if they had an apparently Anglo name but ordered held until trial if they had an apparently Hispanic name.

Type C would be released regardless of their apparent ethnicity.

We are assuming that there is nobody ordered detained because they are Anglo rather than Hispanic; that is, we assume that the ethnic discrimination goes in only one direction. Of course, we can't directly observe the proportions of these latent types in the population, but by randomly labeling a case with an Anglo versus a Hispanic name, we guarantee that the expected proportions of these three latent types must be the same in both ethnic groups. This was the advantage of randomization that was described in chapter 2—that it balances all covariates, even unobserved ones, across the treatment groups. Let's describe these unknown proportions as $P(A)$, $P(B)$, and $P(C)$, respectively. The magnitude of irrational ethnic discrimination,

TABLE 9.1

A randomized trial of assigning apparently Anglo versus Hispanic names to defendants

	Hispanic name group	Anglo name group
	(n = 30)	(n = 30)
Detained	18	6
Released	12	24
Total	30	30

therefore, is simply P(B), the proportion of type B cases in the population, and if this proportion is zero, then the judge is not ethnically biased.

Now we conduct our study with thirty apparently Anglo and thirty apparently Hispanic defendants, and the observed results are presented in table 9.1.

The number who receive an order for pretrial detention in the Hispanic group logically must be P(A) + P(B), whereas the number detained in the Anglo group must be simply P(A). The ratio of these numbers is the causal effect of ethnicity on the judge's decision, and it is:

$$(18/30)/(6/30) = 18/6 = 3.0$$

One could therefore say that the causal effect of Hispanic ethnicity is to *triple* the rate of pretrial detention, holding all background factors constant. And this is indeed how the result will often be reported. But notice that it does not isolate the quantity that we set out to find, which is P(B), the proportion of defendants whose detention is causally attributable to their perceived ethnicity.

Randomization allowed us to identify P(A) + P(B) = 18/30, P(A) = 6/30, and their ratio [P(A) + P(B)]/P(A) = 3.0. But how can we isolate P(B)? Using a ratio measure of disparity, we can't. The obvious solution, however, is to take the difference contrast rather than the ratio contrast. That is, the difference of P(A) + P(B) in the Hispanic group minus P(A) in the Anglo group yields P(B). That yields a total of 18 − 6 = 12 Hispanic defendants who were detained *because of their ethnicity*, a number completely

TABLE 9.2

A randomized trial of assigning apparently Anglo versus Hispanic names to defendants, adding a prior conviction

	Hispanic name group (n = 30)	Anglo name group (n = 30)
Detained	24	8
Released	6	22
Total	30	30

obscured by the relative contrast. The missing quantity P(B) is therefore found as $(18/30) - (6/30) = 12/30 = 0.40$, and thus in 40 percent of the cases we examined, the decision would tip one way or the other depending on the ethnicity of the defendant, a statement that could not be made using the ratio contrast.

But it gets even more interesting. The result obtained above is a function of the distribution of cases we examined. Let's try the same experiment but this time add a prior conviction to every case file that is brought before the judge. Once again, we will use sixty defendants, split between thirty with apparently Hispanic names and thirty with apparently Anglo names; only this time, the judge will opt to detain more of the defendants in light of their criminal backgrounds. The new results are presented in table 9.2.

The ratio $[P(A) + P(B)]/P(A) = (24/30)/(8/30) = 3.0$ reveals that, once again, Hispanic ethnicity has tripled the rate of pretrial detention, and thus it seems that nothing has changed. By now, however, you might start to suspect that the ratio doesn't always tell "the whole truth and nothing but the truth." The difference measure clarifies that $(24/30) - (8/30) = 16/30 = 0.533$, and thus rather than 40 percent of Hispanic defendants being victims of discrimination, the number now is 53.3 percent. The ratio measure told you only that the numerator was triple the denominator, but it never told you what that denominator was or revealed how it changed from the first experiment to the second. In the first experiment, twelve Hispanic defendants were held solely because of their ethnicity because 40 percent of thirty is twelve. In the second experiment, it was 53.3 percent, or sixteen out of the thirty defendants. Thus, four more of the thirty Hispanic individuals were impacted by ethnic discrimination in the second trial than the first, even though the ratio effects remained exactly 3.0 in both studies.[9]

The ratio of risks has another quirk, which is that it is not symmetric. This means that an arbitrary difference in coding a variable can change the number dramatically. For example, suppose we compare the risk of a having stroke among Dutch compared to Bolivians. The risks in each group are 6 percent and 3 percent, respectively. The difference contrast is therefore 3 percent and the ratio is 2.0. No problem. Except why did we have to consider the probability of *having* the stroke instead of the probability of *not having* the stroke? Those are two sides of the same coin, so the disparity in one outcome ought to be the same as the other. The proportions without strokes are 94 percent and 97 percent, respectively. The magnitude of the difference measure between the groups is still the same 3 percent, no matter which direction you choose for the subtraction. But now look what happens to the ratio: $0.94/0.97 = 0.97$ and $0.97/0.94 = 1.03$; so depending on which way you happened to take the contrast, the magnitude has changed dramatically from 2.0 to something very close to 1.0. That's a problem.

Another practical issue is that when investigators have other variables that they need to control for, they want to estimate the disparity using a regression model, and regression models for risk ratios are surprisingly difficult to work with. These models often crash a statistical software program or fail to provide a solution.[10] To solve both the symmetry problem and the estimation problem, a common solution is to use a more convoluted ratio measure, the odds ratio. The odds are calculated as the probability of getting the outcome divided by the probability of not getting it. Odds are commonly encountered in betting contexts, like a racetrack where a horse might have odds of 20 to 1, meaning that you are paid $20 for every $1 bet if your chosen horse wins the race. For people who don't spend a lot of time betting on horses, however, the term *odds* probably has no specific mathematical connotation, and indeed, the word doesn't even exist in most languages other than English.[11]

In the case of the earlier stroke comparison, the odds of stroke for the Dutch are $0.06/0.94 = 0.064$. The odds for the Bolivians are $0.03/0.97 = 0.031$. Therefore, the odds ratio equals $0.064/0.031 = 2.06$. Now switching to the odds of *not* getting a stroke, it would be $0.97/0.03 = 32.33$ in the Bolivians and $0.94/0.06 = 15.67$ in the Dutch, and the odds ratio remains $32.33/15.67 = 2.06$ (table 9.3). Bingo. The odds ratio here is perfectly symmetric. It also has the nice mathematical property that it is very easy to

TABLE 9.3

Calculating various measures for the disparity in stroke between Dutch and Bolivians

	Stroke	No stroke
Dutch	$\dfrac{6}{100}$	$\dfrac{94}{100}$
Bolivians	$\dfrac{3}{100}$	$\dfrac{97}{100}$
Risk difference	$\left(\dfrac{6}{100}-\dfrac{3}{100}\right)=\dfrac{3}{100}$	$\left(\dfrac{97}{100}-\dfrac{94}{100}\right)=\dfrac{3}{100}$
Risk ratio	$\left(\dfrac{6}{100}\Big/\dfrac{3}{100}\right)=2.0$	$\left(\dfrac{97}{100}\Big/\dfrac{94}{100}\right)=1.03$
Odds ratio	$\dfrac{\left(\dfrac{6}{100}\Big/\dfrac{94}{100}\right)}{\left(\dfrac{3}{100}\Big/\dfrac{97}{100}\right)}=\dfrac{0.064}{0.031}=2.06$	$\dfrac{\left(\dfrac{97}{100}\Big/\dfrac{3}{100}\right)}{\left(\dfrac{94}{100}\Big/\dfrac{6}{100}\right)}=\dfrac{32.22}{15.67}=2.06$

model with something called *logistic regression*, and this has become the workhorse of quantitative biomedicine and social sciences for these reasons.

There's always a catch, however. And for the odds ratio, probably the biggest problem is simply that almost nobody without a PhD in statistics knows what the hell it means. Obviously, it is a ratio of two odds, and each of these odds is itself a ratio of two probabilities, the outcome happening versus the outcome not happening. It's not rocket science, but what I mean is that most people don't have very good intuitions about its magnitude. And because the calculation is so convoluted, they tend to simply interpret it like the ratio of the risks, which it is not. When the outcome is relatively unlikely, as in our stroke example, this is not far off (2.0 versus 2.06). But as the outcome becomes more common, it can exaggerate the effect size, sometimes dramatically.[12]

The last few paragraphs were thick with statistical issues, so I need to demonstrate that these are consequential problems for the real-world study of racial and ethnic disparities. To make this case, let's turn to a famous experimental study conducted to investigate clinical biases by race and sex through the "audit study" design that was described in chapter 2. In 1999, health economist Kevin Schulman and colleagues developed a computerized survey to assess 720 physicians managing chest pain as described to them by one of eight videotaped actors reading an identical script. The actors were white or Black, men or women, and the investigators focused on the roles of race and gender on the recommendations provided, controlling for other factors such as age.[13] The authors published their results in the *New England Journal of Medicine*, reporting that women (odds ratio = 0.6) and Blacks (odds ratio = 0.6) were less likely to be referred for cardiac catheterization than men and whites, respectively. Considering both gender and race together, they noted that Black women were less likely to be referred for catheterization than white men (odds ratio = 0.4). Recall that this odds ratio of 0.4 means that the odds of referral for Black women are only 40 percent as large as the odds of referral for white men, where the odds are defined as the probability of being referred divided by the probability of not being referred.

The study captured considerable media attention, with headline news coverage from major television networks and a response from the U.S. surgeon general on the ABC evening news show *Nightline*.[14] Across newspaper and television platforms, the media consistently misinterpreted the odds ratio. For example, *USA Today* wrote, "Blacks and women with chest pain are 40 percent less likely than whites or men to be referred by physicians for cardiac catheterization."[15] Other major media outlets wrote pretty much the same thing. But recall that it is the odds that are 40 percent lower, not the probabilities. As I noted earlier, ratio measures hide information and odds ratios are particularly difficult for readers to understand. The reported odds ratio for the Black actors was 0.6, and this measure is formed by the odds of referral for Blacks divided by the odds of referral for whites. What were these odds? Back-calculating from the referral rates, we find that these were 84.7/15.3 = 5.5 and 90.6/9.4 = 9.6, so that 5.5/9.6 = 0.6. Because the proportions referred were actually 84.7 and 90.6 for Blacks and whites, respectively, the risk ratio is actually a much more modest value of 0.9. What the news media should have reported is that Blacks and women with chest pain are *10 percent* less likely than whites or men to be referred, not *40 percent* less likely. The problem is that most decisions were to refer the "patient" for screening, and so the prevalence of the outcome was very high. In this circumstance, the odds are much larger than the risks. Because most journalists and lay readers

TABLE 9.4

Expressing a disparity as a ratio of proportions

	Referred	Not referred
Black	847	153
White	906	94
Ratio of proportions	$\left(\dfrac{847}{1,000} \Big/ \dfrac{906}{1,000}\right) = 0.935$	$\left(\dfrac{153}{1,000} \Big/ \dfrac{94}{1,000}\right) = 0.614$

have no idea what an odds ratio is, they naturally fall back on the risk-ratio interpretation, which in this setting was dramatically mistaken.

In fact, there are various options available to researchers, and it's not always easy to know what is the best contrast to make. Suppose we study a thousand people and come up with results like those in the Schulman paper:

Blacks: 847 referred, 153 not referred (84.7 percent referred)
Whites: 906 referred, 94 not referred (90.6 percent referred)

There seem to be at least four natural choices for contrasts one could make: (1) the ratio of proportions (risk ratio); (2) the ratio of odds (odds ratio); (3) the difference between proportions (risk difference); and (4) the reciprocal of difference between proportions. All are mathematically legitimate, and each has advantages and disadvantages. No single one is a slam dunk.

First let's take the ratio of proportions. This is easy for readers to understand. But in this example, it can be either 0.935 (if the proportions referred are contrasted) or 0.614 (if the proportions not referred are contrasted), differing because of the lack of symmetry that was noted earlier (table 9.4). Therefore, an author would have to make some case for choosing one over the other, and people may disagree over this choice. And as mentioned earlier, it's technically challenging to fit a regression model for this contrast with adjustment for confounders.

Second, let's take the odds ratio. For these numbers, as we have seen, it is 0.57 (which was previously rounded to 0.6), and it is very far from the ratio of proportions (table 9.5). Journalists and lay readers will confuse these, and the predictable result is that most readers will understand the effect magnitude

TABLE 9.5
Expressing a disparity as an odds ratio

	Referred	Not referred
Black	847	153
White	906	94

Odds ratio

$$\dfrac{\left(\dfrac{847}{1,000} \Big/ \dfrac{153}{1,000}\right)}{\left(\dfrac{906}{1,000} \Big/ \dfrac{94}{1,000}\right)} = \dfrac{5.54}{9.64} = 0.57 \qquad \dfrac{\left(\dfrac{94}{1,000} \Big/ \dfrac{906}{1,000}\right)}{\left(\dfrac{153}{1,000} \Big/ \dfrac{847}{1,000}\right)} = \dfrac{0.104}{0.180} = 0.57$$

to be much larger than it actually is. I showed earlier how the risk ratio mis-states the causal effect of a treatment, and the odds ratio is even worse in this regard because it will change its value with adjustment for covariates even if these covariates are not confounders.[16] On the plus side, however, the odds ratio is symmetric, so one no longer has to make a case for studying referral versus nonreferral as the outcome. And it's extremely easy to estimate from a regression model with covariate adjustments, even though the interpretation of the adjusted odds ratio can become substantially more difficult.

Third, let's look at the difference of proportions. This has the same absolute magnitude (5.9 per 100 patients) whether contrasting proportions referred or proportions not referred (table 9.6). Given the advantages described ear-lier with respect to transparency, symmetry, and the direct translation into statements about affected individuals, it seems to beat all the ratios. But once again, it is more difficult to estimate from a regression model if covariate

TABLE 9.6
Expressing a disparity as a difference of proportions

	Referred	Not referred
Black	847	153
White	906	94

Difference of proportions

$$\left(\dfrac{906}{1,000} - \dfrac{847}{1,000}\right) = 0.059 \qquad \left(\dfrac{153}{1,000} - \dfrac{94}{1,000}\right) = 0.059$$

adjustment is needed. Economists will generally manage this quite easily with an ordinary linear model for the probability. Most biostatisticians find this model abhorrent, however, so it remains rare to handle it that way in biomedical applications.[17]

Finally, there is the option of taking the reciprocal of the difference between proportions, where the reciprocal of a number refers to taking one divided by that number. For example, the reciprocal of 0.05 is $\frac{1}{0.05} = 20$. This is a very popular transformation for the difference between proportions because it expresses the number of subjects required in the group with the lower rate of adverse outcomes to prevent one such outcome. For this reason, clinical epidemiologists refer to this measure as the *number needed to treat* (NNT).[18] Suppose we conduct a randomized trial of a pill for reducing incidence of toenail fungus, and the proportions affected at the end of the trial are 5 percent among those taking the pill and 10 percent among those taking a placebo. In that case, the difference of proportions is 0.05, and the NNT equals $1/0.05 = 20$, which means that a doctor must give this pill to twenty people to prevent one case. When being Black or white is a modifiable aspect of the information presented to a judge, as it is in the audit design where doctors can be shown one actor or the other, then this contrast reveals that having $1/0.059 = 17$ people in the white group generates one additional referral, due to the higher white rate. Or if referrals are regarded as undesirable (as they might be from the point of view of the insurance company), having seventeen people in the Black group would prevent one referral, due to the lower Black rate. The advantage of taking the reciprocal of the difference is to express the impact in terms of the number of whole patients whose status will be changed.

Interpreting race or ethnicity as a "treatment" with a contrast like the NNT might seem strange at first, but I think it comes closest to the normative ethical intuitions underlying tort law and other systems for assessing harms to individuals. People experience death, disease, and other adverse outcomes as whole individuals, whereas risks deal with fractions of populations. To know that you are in a group that has 63 percent higher risk of missing out on a referral is too abstract. It has no anchor to quantifiable harms to you, the individual human being. The absolute risk of 0.059 is better, but people do not experience risks; they experience events. This absolute risk of 0.059 can therefore be directly translated into fifty-nine excess nonreferrals per thousand people "treated" to this higher rate. To take the reciprocal of this risk as $\frac{1,000}{59}$ expresses these excess cases as one for every seventeen so exposed. This is just another way to make it even more concrete—to show an actual body count.

This advantage of absolute risks and NNTs is especially clear when assessing the harmful impacts of racial and ethnic disparities and reinforces how misleading the ratio measures can be when one wants to know where the harm is greatest. Consider a study by the physician Stacey Jolley and colleagues on cardiovascular disease prevalence and mortality among Blacks compared to whites in the United States.[19] The authors considered the age pattern of this racial inequality, reporting that the largest Black-white disparities were observed in relatively younger individuals, and therefore the authors argued that reducing racial disparities required a particular focus of resources on young and middle-aged Black Americans to have the greatest impact. This conclusion rested on the observation that among people between the ages of thirty-five and forty-four, cardiovascular disease prevalence was almost twice as high among Blacks than among whites and that this ratio decreased with each decade, narrowing to a 20 percent excess for those between sixty-five and seventy-four and finally to roughly equal prevalences for those age seventy-five and older.

With respect to where the greatest harm is done to individuals, this is completely backward of course. The striking pattern of diminishing harms with age emerges as a statistical artifact of the authors' arbitrary decision to report the relative contrasts rather than the absolute contrasts. Those between thirty-five and forty-four years old have a prevalence difference of 1,759 per 100,000 population, which grows to 2,071 among those forty-five to fifty-four and to 5,399 among those fifty-five to sixty-four, thereafter falling again. Inverting these like NNTs, we find that among the young, there is one excess case of prevalent cardiovascular disease for every fifty-seven Black Americans (100,000/1,759), where "excess" refers to the number of existing cases in excess of what they would have been if they enjoyed the lower white prevalence. This rises to an excess case in every forty-eight Black Americans (100,000/2,071) in the next decade, and further still to one in every eighteen (100,000/5,399) among those ages fifty-five to sixty-four (figure 9.2). If you prefer, one extra case per eighteen is a little more than five extra prevalent cases per one hundred. Both of these are functions of the absolute difference, not the unitless prevalence ratio. And they both show that the harm to the greatest number of individuals happens for those age fifty-five to sixty-four and not the younger adults as stated in the published paper.

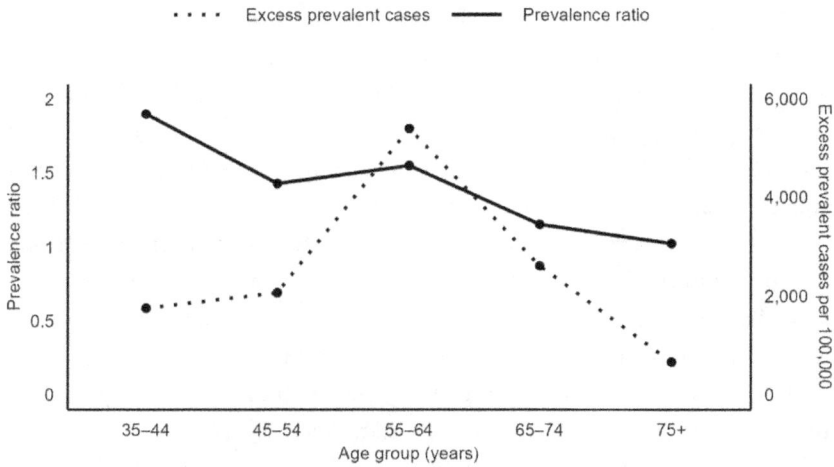

Figure 9.2 Disparity in prevalent cardiovascular disease by race.

Source: Stacey Jolly et al., "Higher Cardiovascular Disease Prevalence and Mortality Among Younger Blacks Compared to Whites," *American Journal of Medicine* 123, no. 9 (2010): 811–18.

Taking this calculation one step further, these absolute effect contrasts are expressed per 100,000 people, but they ignore how many people we are really talking about in each age and race category in the U.S. population. In the 2000 census, which is the closest census to the data included in this paper, people between the ages of thirty-five and forty-four made up approximately 16 percent of the Black population, whereas those between the ages of fifty-five and sixty-four were slightly less than 7 percent. This suggests that the excess Black prevalence was actually about 97,000 cases for the younger group versus 128,000 for the older group. The burden for the younger group is still smaller, but the numbers are much closer given the age structure of the population. If you then consider that younger people have more years of life affected by a chronic condition or may lose more potential years of life by dying prematurely, the young group could be the more affected after all.[20] This shows not only how complicated it can be to answer a simple question about where a disparity is most acute but also how important it is to consider the age structure of the population as a real feature driving disparities experienced by individuals, contrary to the reflexive age adjustment to an arbitrary standard that was discussed in chapter 3.

Yet another interesting wrinkle to point out is about the exaggeration of the effect magnitude by the odds ratio that was demonstrated in the Schulman study. This exaggeration occurs when we compare one group to another group, such as the odds of referral in one racial group contrasted with the odds of referral in another racial group, where these are nonoverlapping groups. There is an interesting exception worth noting, which is that the crude odds ratio could in fact be better in situations where one group is compared to the entire population to detect differential treatment, in which case the interpretation can become much more intuitive (as long as there is no further adjustment). An example of this is the legal question of whether Black drivers are stopped by police disproportionately to their representation in the population. The statistician Joseph Kadane recounts a legal case in New Jersey from 1996 in which county public defenders moved on behalf of seventeen defendants to have evidence against them dismissed on grounds of differential enforcement.[21] The concern arose over searches of the clients' cars on the New Jersey turnpike, and the public defenders gathered data from police records demonstrating that in a relevant time window, 46.2 percent of the drivers stopped by the New Jersey State Police were Black, whereas observations conducted by the public defenders revealed that only 15 percent of turnpike drivers were Black. Kadane then shows that one can construct an odds ratio as the odds of being Black if stopped divided by the odds of being Black in the whole population. With some algebra, this eventually reduces to the proportion stopped if Black divided by the proportion stopped if not Black.[22] In this specific court case, the numbers above were expressed as the odds ratio, which was ($[0.462/0.15]/[0.538/0.85]$) = 4.86. This can be directly interpreted as Black drivers being almost five times more likely to be stopped, a measure that was used by the judge in his decision and accepted as the relevant measure by both parties.

The ongoing documentation of racial and ethnic disparities by government agencies and academic researchers is a vital effort and provides the evidence base for understanding how these differences arise and what can be done to ameliorate them. As we saw in the traffic stop example, examining disparities is essential to reveal and combat discriminatory treatment. But as this chapter has shown, this process is not entirely straightforward. There are many choices that must be made, and here we focused on the choices around effect contrast scales and measures. Unfortunately, the prevailing situation in most countries is that the ratio scale contrast takes priority, despite its many deficiencies noted earlier. Especially in academic work, this scale is often pursued by using the odds ratio measure, which can lead to even more difficulties in interpretation across researchers, journalists, policymakers, and the public. Indeed, there are even more obscure measures that are often used, such as hazard ratios in time-to-event studies, and so the situation can get even more convoluted.

One particularly hostile reaction to this cacophony of scales, measures, and misinterpretations is to declare that, as a society, we simply do not know how to document disparities at all.[23] The attorney James Scanlan has written a number of essays to this effect, casting doubt on the whole complex infrastructure of disparities monitoring over these apparent contradictions. In particular, he notes a sort of homeopathic paradox in disparities research, in which the measure of disparity appears to grow as the adverse condition is titrated down to zero prevalence (figure 9.3).[24] This is premised on a ratio measure of disparities, of course. Imagine two racial or ethnic groups with different rates of tuberculosis, as in the paper discussed earlier in this chapter, and imagine that we gradually but steadily eliminate tuberculosis from all groups in the population. The advantaged group will have a rate approaching zero over time, and as it gets ever closer to zero, the ratio formed by dividing by this denominator will explode to larger and larger values. Mathematical readers will note that in the limit as the

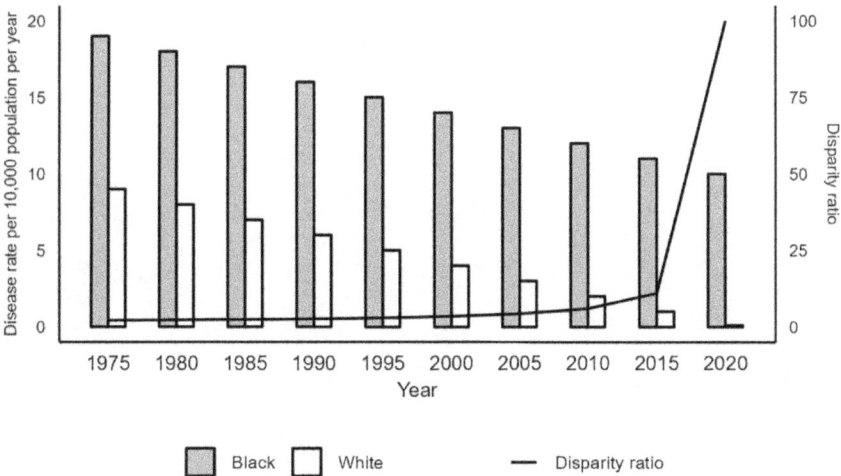

Figure 9.3 The homeopathic paradox.

denominator of a ratio goes to zero, the ratio goes to infinity. Therefore, according to Scanlan's critique, we must experience nearly infinitely large disparities before we can eliminate any bad outcomes from the population, and the closer we get to ridding ourselves of undesirable things like diseases, the worse the disparities will appear.[25]

Let's not throw the baby out with the bathwater. It is true that this is tricky territory, but that doesn't mean it shouldn't be done or that it can't be done better. If we don't even try to monitor disparities, we have no quantitative basis on which to assess social progress toward racial justice. Scanlon's critique derives largely from the dominance of ratio measures, and indeed, it appears that these are overemphasized across a wide range of disciplines. This should change, but that is only a start toward a more diligent, comprehensive, and thoughtful documentation of inequalities. This chapter only scratches the surface of this topic, and many technical publications pursue these measures more exhaustively.[26] This is not simply a mathematical exercise. Instead, it's a necessary decision that involves ethical judgements and consideration of trade-offs, as different values are represented by these competing measures. In this sense, there will never be a single objective approach to quantification of racial and ethnic disparities but always a range of options, each providing a slightly different perspective.

CHAPTER X

What Explains a Disparity?

How do we reveal the mechanism that *explains* an incident event? Given some potential causal paths, a logical approach might be to shut down one path and see if this blocks the event from occurring. Say I leave a cookie on the kitchen table each night, and the next morning I always find it missing. I have only two hypotheses for this disappearance: the dog or the children. Clearly I must disable one of these pathways to find out which one is to blame. To avoid falling afoul of Child Protective Services, I decide that it is the dog who will spend the night locked in a crate. In the morning, when I find that the cookie has still disappeared, the dog is exonerated, and a shadow of heavy suspicion falls onto the children.

Scientists, using experiments, engage in much the same strategy to identify causal pathways, shutting down all but one chain of sequential causes to see which one is the explanation for a phenomenon of interest. It is no surprise, therefore, that statisticians mimic this same logic with their models, shutting down pathways with statistical adjustments to test explanatory hypotheses.

In previous chapters, we discussed the use of statistical adjustments to combat biases such as confounding and selection, but there is also the common practice of using adjustments to mimic an experiment, like the previous cookie example, in which some potential pathways are blocked to distinguish their contributions to the overall effect. In fact, the adjustment for a confounder can also be described this way, if you recall from chapter 4 confounding involves a confusion between two explanatory paths connecting the treatment to the outcome, one of which is shut down by the adjustment. But these pathways being disabled in confounder adjustments are what Judea Pearl calls "backdoor" pathways because they are pathways that lead into the treatment. When instead the pathway being shut down is one coming out of the treatment, the analysis is referred to as *mediation* or *effect decomposition*, depending on the discipline.[1] This statistical approach is also widely used in the study of racial and ethnic disparities. After all, there are rarely variables in the dataset that have pathways leading *into* race or ethnicity, by which we mean quantities that are causes of these identities. However, many variables are affected by race and ethnicity, so there are many pathways flowing out from race and ethnicity.

In all the previously described adjustments for various study biases, we carefully avoided adjusting for anything that was itself affected by the treatment. This is because the causal effect of interest is the contrast between setting a population to be treated versus setting that same population to be untreated, and so if one were to manipulate a quantity downstream from that treatment, it would interfere with the very effect we hope to estimate. For example, suppose we want to know the effect of a new policy that adds a $1 tax to the sale price of each package of cigarettes. The outcome is the population incidence of heart attacks. Our dataset has one measured covariate available, which is the number of cigarettes consumed each year per capita, and the causal structure of the data-generating process looks like that shown in figure 10.1.

If we are interested in the causal impact of this policy on the heart attack rate, would it be wise to adjust statistically for the number of cigarettes smoked? Absolutely not! The reason is that the one mechanism by which the law has its effect is exactly by reducing the consumption of cigarettes. Holding this variable constant changes the question to a comparison of two

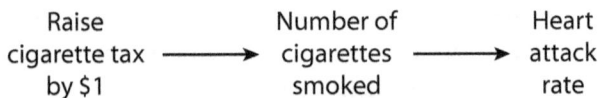

Raise cigarette tax by $1 ⟶ Number of cigarettes smoked ⟶ Heart attack rate

Figure 10.1 Hypothesized causal relationship between an increase in cigarette prices, number of cigarettes smoked, and rate of heart attacks.

groups that smoke exactly the same amount, even though one group pays more to do so. Because the tax policy effect is *mediated* by the volume of cigarettes consumed, holding this constant will completely block the effect. In the adjusted analysis, the effect will be determined to be null, and yet this is false—the true effect of the policy is to lower the heart attack rate.[2] A bias arises in the adjusted analysis because the one relevant pathway has been shut down by the adjustment. Think of mediation like a game of dominoes. The first domino tumbles and hits the second, which tumbles into the third. To adjust for the middle domino, holding it constant, is to catch it from falling onto the next domino, so we cannot see how the action is transmitted from the first domino to the last. Intervening or adjusting for the mediator therefore interrupts the causal chain, disabling the causal effect of the treatment.

We are rather confident that simply paying more for cigarettes does not modify their pathological potential. But suppose we change to an example with more than one causal pathway potentially operating. Consider a trial of a smoking cessation program, where the outcome is again incident heart attack and the mediator is a person's cholesterol level (figure 10.2).[3]

Now when we intervene to change someone from a smoker to a non-smoker through the intervention, this lowers the person's cholesterol value, which in turn lowers their heart attack risk—like a chain of falling dominos. But there may be another pathway as well because cholesterol might not be the only downstream physiological change precipitated by smoking cessation. We refer to the path through cholesterol as the "indirect path" because it is mediated by a quantity that is salient to us, and we refer to the other pathway as a "direct path" because it is not mediated by any variables that we have measured and included in the analysis. Of course, the direct path also operates through discrete physiological steps, even if we don't happen to know exactly what they are. In an actual experiment, we would set the smoking level by applying the cessation program or not and set the cholesterol level to low (by giving statins) or high (by making the person spend

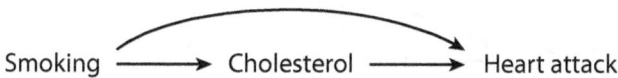

Smoking ⟶ Cholesterol ⟶ Heart attack

Figure 10.2 Hypothesized causal relationship between smoking cessation, serum cholesterol, and incident heart attack showing direct and indirect effects.

a year living in France). The magnitude of the smoking cessation effect observed while holding cholesterol constant would be the direct effect of smoking, and the direct effect would differ from the total effect if there is also an indirect effect relayed through changes to cholesterol.

Rather than running real experiments, social science and disparities researchers generally fit statistical models to observed data, and in this context, statistical control stands in for the physical control described earlier. The fitting and interpretation of these statistical models are complex topics with many technical details, assumptions, and caveats, but in broad outline, there are two general flavors of mediated effect that one can estimate. The first are *controlled effects*, which correspond to the imagined intervention of fixing the mediator to one specific value for everyone. The other type are *natural effects* (which earlier authors referred to as *pure effects*).[4] These hold the mediator to the value that would have occurred naturally at some reference level of the treatment. Natural effects have been interpreted by Judea Pearl as reflecting a "disabling" of the arrow between treatment and mediator.[5] In 2014, the biostatistician Tyler VanderWeele and the epidemiologist Whitney Robinson provided a comprehensive formalization of these methods specifically for the problem of explaining racial and ethnic disparities.[6] The major innovation in that paper was to consider the descriptive racial or ethnic disparity as the quantity being decomposed, rather than a causal effect of treatment in the counterfactual sense. This means that there is no imagined swapping of racial or ethnic categories, only the question of how the observed disparity would change with potential interventions to the mediating variable or variables.

VanderWeele and Robinson's setup allows us to ask what proportion of an overall racial or ethnic disparity is relayed through some set of specific material, psychological, or behavioral intermediates. For example, consider race, income, and mortality (figure 10.3).

We know that one's racial classification from birth affects life chances for educational and occupational opportunities and that these in turn affect

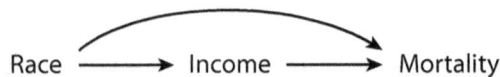

Race ⟶ Income ⟶ Mortality

Figure 10.3 Hypothesized causal relationship between race, income, and mortality showing direct and indirect effects.

mortality rates. We can therefore posit a causal chain through a measured intermediate like income. Of course, there are other pathways, like living in a better or worse neighborhood, and these all fall on the direct pathway in figure 10.3. The controlled effects in the figure correspond to the disparity that would be observed if we were to assign a single income level to everyone, but this may not be an especially useful model. It seems weird enough to assign incomes to people, but it is especially unrealistic that everyone would have the same value. Natural effects thus seem much more, well, natural. VanderWeele and Robinson proposed that if we are interested in the disparity between Blacks and whites, then we take the advantaged group as the referent and assign to each Black person a randomly drawn income from the white distribution.[7] Under this hypothetical intervention, therefore, Blacks and whites end up with the same distribution of incomes: the same average and the same spread of values around the average. This corresponds nicely with Pearl's account of "disabling" the arrow from race to income. Indeed, if we imagine a world without racial discrimination, it is exactly the world in which income is not a function of racial classification.[8] Then the total racial disparity based on real-world incomes can be contrasted with the modeled racial disparity that would be observed if the arrow from race were disabled, and the difference between these two racial disparities is the portion that is mediated by income or, put another way, explained by income.

Long before this modern statistical approach was formalized, an ad hoc version was commonly applied to seek nature-versus-nurture explanations for health disparities by including some measured covariates as intermediates and declaring any remaining direct effect to be evidence of a genetic explanation. This is illogical, of course, because unmeasured causes of the disparity could just as easily be social or behavioral as genetic, but this strategy nonetheless dominated medical journals in the 1980s and 1990s. As a classic example of this genre of paper, consider a highly cited 1992 *JAMA* paper by the clinical researcher Frederick Brancati and his colleagues that sought to explain Black excess incidence of diabetic end-stage renal disease (ESRD).[9] The authors had data from a statewide ESRD registry covering more than two million adults along with ecological data from household risk factor surveys at the ZIP-code level. Black residents were found to have a 3.42-fold higher incidence of the disease, as well as a higher prevalence of many of its risk factors, including diabetes, hypertension, and lower educational attainment. After adjusting for these measured clinical risk factors and the education measure, the adjusted racial disparity was reduced to a

2.70-fold higher incidence. The authors therefore concluded that excess incidence of diabetic ESRD in Blacks was not due to racial differences in age, socioeconomic status, or access to healthcare and, therefore, must have been due to "an inheritable genetic predisposition."[10]

The statistical logic here is a kind of process of elimination: if it's not due to the things we measured, it must be due to the things we didn't measure. It's like the famous Sherlock Holmes quote that once you eliminate the impossible, then whatever remains must be true, even if improbable.[11] But there is a rather striking elision in this example between adjustment for a member of a set and adjusting for the whole set. To state that one has adjusted for apples doesn't imply that one has adjusted for all fruits. In this paper, the authors adjust for education and then conclude that the difference cannot be attributed to socioeconomic status, but the latter is certainly much broader than education. Moreover, the authors didn't even really have educational information on individuals. What they actually knew was the address of each person, which they connected to survey data at the ZIP-code level on the proportion of residents who had at least some post-secondary education. The analysis therefore rests on the following premise: that a Black and white person who each reside in a ZIP code that has the same proportion of people who went to college would themselves share the same socioeconomic status. Based on this statistical control, the authors declared that the alternate hypothesis of socioeconomic inequality had been addressed and dismissed and so the cause must lie elsewhere. And of all the near-infinite number of things that are not adjusted for in this model, they somehow conclude that the explanation can only be a genetic factor.[12]

Alas, this was the state of biomedical research on racial and ethnic disparities circa 1992, but we've come a long way since then. In particular, with the advent of the Human Genome Project, it became passé to speculate about vague genetic factors because actual genotype measures had become available. Moreover, we've since clarified the assumptions and potential biases inherent in the mediation model, including the realization that any measurement error or misspecification of the indirect effect naturally inflates the direct effect.[13] Therefore, if I adjust for apples on the indirect pathway, all the other fruit ends up on the direct pathway. Even though we know better now, it's still good to be wary of this sleight of hand, which still pops up now and then in the scientific literature and even more so in popular discourse. For example, in 2018, there was a highly publicized debate between authors Sam Harris and Ezra Klein on racial differences in intelligence. Harris's position, echoing work by the political scientist Charles Murray, was that there must be a genetic difference between groups because the racial difference in measured intelligence persists despite adjustment for some measures of differential social environment.[14] This was the crux of the argument in Murray's 1994 book with Richard Herrnstein, *The Bell Curve*, which remains the definitive statement of this thesis.[15] Many scholars have criticized the book based on these fallacious statistical arguments,[16] but the passionate defense of Murray's work by Harris just a few years ago speaks to the relentless persistence of this erroneous statistical inference.

Trying to use a mediation model to solve the old nature-versus-nurture question seems doomed because one could never hope to shut down all of the paths for either domain. Our knowledge of the pathways for genes and environments—not to mention how they interact—is still far too incomplete. The premise of the 1992 *JAMA* paper and the 1994 book by Herrnstein and Murray was clearly that because the indirect pathway through social differences was controlled, any remaining difference must be innate, presumably genetic. But potential social differences are near infinite and notoriously difficult to measure, making the prospect of shutting down this pathway rather absurd. Therefore, mediation of a racial or ethnic disparity seems much more credible when the mediator is instead a well-defined and well-measured quantity that represents a plausible explanation for the observed disparity.

To illustrate a more tractable hypothesis along these lines, consider a recent paper in the *American Journal of Epidemiology*.[17] The clinical researcher Melissa Bartick and colleagues were interested in the racial and ethnic disparity observed in sudden unexpected infant death (SUID), for which non-Hispanic Black and American Indian/Alaskan Native infants are disproportionately affected. These groups have roughly 40 percent higher odds of SUID, adjusted for other covariates. The authors noted that these groups also exhibit lower rates of breastfeeding and wanted to determine what proportion of the SUID disparity might be explained by this breastfeeding deficit. They aimed to estimate the natural direct and indirect effects, which is to say the contrast in outcomes if racial and ethnic minorities were to breastfeed at the same rate as the white participants. They had data on more than thirteen million live births and about twelve thousand SUID death certificates from the United States between 2015 and 2018. Overall, not breastfeeding was associated with a 14 percent excess odds of SUID, or roughly one extra SUID for every ten thousand live births. But despite the dominos

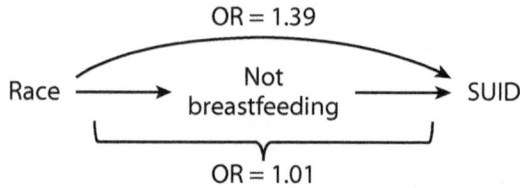

OR = 1.39

Race → Not breastfeeding → SUID

OR = 1.01

Total disparity Black versus white, OR = 1.40
Disparity when Black breastfeeding set equal to white breastfeeding, OR = 1.39
Proportion of racial disparity explained by breastfeeding = 2.3%

Figure 10.4 Mediation of excess sudden unexpected infant death among Blacks via less breastfeeding compared to whites, United States, 2015–2018.

Source: Melissa Bartick et al., "The Role of Breastfeeding in Racial and Ethnic Disparities in Sudden Unexpected Infant Death: A Population-Based Study of 13 Million Infants in the United States," *American Journal of Epidemiology* 191, no. 7 (2022): 1190–201.

being lined up as expected, the extent to which breastfeeding disparities explained the SUID disparities turned out to be trivial; roughly 2 percent of the racial disparity would be eliminated if we had all groups breastfeed at the same rate as whites (figure 10.4). Therefore, 98 percent of the gap must be due to other exposures or behaviors that were not measured in this study.

This sudden infant death paper is a more sensible example of a modern application of this technique, but it's still important to recognize that the causal interpretation of these models remains rather fragile even when, as in this example, the mediator is more clearly defined. This is because the identification of the natural effect rests on a lot of assumptions, and if considered closely, these assumptions might not seem very plausible. The controlled direct effect could be obtained in an actual randomized trial, and this estimate would be much more secure because randomization would obviate any concerns about unmeasured confounders. It might seem surprising or even unethical to randomize women to breastfeeding, but this has actually been done in large trials by simply randomizing women to receive extra support and encouragement to breastfeed, thereby nudging some women into treatment while having no effect on the women who are resolute in their prior commitment to breastfeed or not breastfeed.[18] The resulting causal inference is then restricted to the subset of women who would be impacted by such a nudge, which is referred to in the literature as the "complier" stratum. Many statistical techniques, for example instrumental variables in economics, similarly restrict inference to the complier subpopulation.[19]

The model in the breastfeeding article would therefore have a good analogy in the concrete world of real experiments had the authors estimated a controlled direct effect. But Bartick and colleagues estimated instead the *natural* direct and indirect effects, and these are more elusive. Presumably this represents a contrast for each minority woman between her observed breastfeeding behavior and the behavior she would have exhibited if she had been white, but this counterfactual is obscure for all of the philosophical and practical reasons reviewed in chapters 2 and 3. Moreover, the authors adjusted for a plethora of covariates, including maternal education, obesity, and insurance status, and one could argue that these might all have likewise been affected by changing the race of the mother.[20] In a traditional treatment effect scenario, we need only believe that there are no unmeasured common causes of the treatment and the outcome. But for estimating the natural direct and indirect effects, we need for there to be no unmeasured common causes of the treatment and outcome, of the treatment and mediator, and of the mediator and outcome. That means the analysis reported here assumed there were no confounders three times over instead of once, which is a lot to assume.

Mediation analyses have long been a workhorse of psychology and sociology and are now increasingly popular in biomedical sciences as well, albeit with varying degrees of technical explanation or justification. It would probably not be an exaggeration to state that, compared to other forms of statistical analysis that are more straightforward and familiar, mediation analyses are much more likely to be conducted poorly. Many authors are vague about whether they are estimating controlled or natural contrasts and seem unsure about the assumptions they are relying on. When reporting adjusted racial or ethnic disparities, there is seldom any discussion of the conceptual dilemmas around racial counterfactuals, which the VanderWeele and Robinson 2014 article sought to resolve. Specifically, those authors promoted the strategy of randomly allocating mediator values from the advantaged group to the disadvantaged group as a way of overcoming the problem of adjusting for covariates affected by race or ethnicity, but this advice has largely been ignored in practice.

Instead, the most common approach still seems to be simply adding the mediator to a standard regression model and reporting the adjusted association as the direct effect.[21] This can be a legitimate way to obtain a controlled direct effect, but it presents several limitations. One is that it assumes that the controlled direct effect is the same across the levels of the mediator. For example, think of the earlier example about the racial disparity in SUID that is potentially mediated by breastfeeding. In a trial, I could theoretically eliminate variability in the mediator either by setting everyone to breastfeed or by setting everyone to not breastfeed, even if the latter might pose some ethical quandaries. The controlled direct effect that I would obtain by simply adding a binary breastfeeding variable to a regression model is the one in which this treatment is held constant at *either* level, meaning that to report a single number as the effect, I must assume that these two disparities are the same. If the disparity happened to be different when everyone breastfeeds compared to what the disparity would be if no one breastfed, then my modeled estimate would lack any clear causal interpretation because it is formed as the hodgepodge of the two distinct effect magnitudes. To emphasize this principle that one should not summarize over heterogeneous values, I often remind students that the man who sleeps with his head in an oven and his feet in a freezer does not feel just fine, on average. Worse, as discussed in chapter 9, these values must necessarily differ on some scale, so that if they happen to be the same on the difference scale, the ratios must differ, and vice versa. Once again, we see that this inference is very fragile.

A more fundamental problem with the notion of controlled direct effects is the idea that a total effect can be decomposed into two parts that are direct and indirect and that these two parts should add up to the whole. This is frequently how such models are interpreted in the literature; so if the controlled direct effect is only half as big as the total effect, then the other half is presumed to be indirect. But this facile interpretation follows from the homogeneity assumption described earlier, which is that the disparity that would be observed when fixing everyone to have the mediator turned on is the same disparity as fixing everyone to have the mediator turned off. This won't generally be true in practice, and the reason it won't be true is that treatments *interact*. What interaction means in this context is that for any two treatments A and B, the causal effect of treatment A might not be the same across the levels of treatment B. For example, a famous study in the late 1970s demonstrated that smoking increased the risk of lung cancer by about tenfold, asbestos increased the risk by about fivefold, and the two exposures together increased the risk by about fiftyfold compared to people without either exposure.[22]

Because of this sort of synergism between treatments, it is entirely possible that the controlled direct effect, which is that part of the total effect that does not flow through the mediator, can actually be larger than the total effect.[23] How could this happen? Consider the following hypothetical example. Suppose that we are interested in the racial disparity ($X = 1$ for

Race ⟶ Unemployment ⟶ Homelessness
(X)   (Z)   (Y)

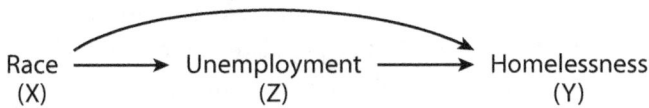

Figure 10.5 Example of relationships between race, unemployment, and homelessness to demonstrate the impact of exposure-mediator interaction.

aboriginal, X = 0 for white) in homelessness (Y = 1 for homeless, Y = 0 otherwise). The mediator is employment status (Z = 1 for unemployed, Z = 0 otherwise) (figure 10.5).

Our task is to consider the proportion of the total racial disparity in homelessness that is attributable to unemployment differences between groups, often expressed as the extent to which unemployment *mediates* the disparity in homelessness. If 100 percent of the disparity is due to unemployment differences between groups, then fixing the same employment status for all individuals (the controlled direct effect) should make the disparity disappear entirely. Alternatively, if 0 percent of the disparity is due to unemployment differences between groups, then fixing the same employment status for all individuals should lead to no change in the disparity whatsoever. Finally, if the disparity diminishes by 50 percent when unemployment is adjusted for in the model, most people would tend to conclude that unemployment differences account for half of the disparity. This is the usual setup, but as we'll see, it doesn't work out very well.

Take a sample of disadvantaged men going through a financial crisis, in which these men have the following counterfactual responses to the mediator:

(a) No matter which racial group they belong to, in the absence of any social intervention, they will become unemployed (Z = 1).
(b) No matter which racial group they belong to, if they become unemployed (Z = 1), they will experience homelessness (Y = 1).
(c) For white men, if assisted through job training and placement (Z = 0), then they will avoid becoming homeless (Y = 0).
(d) For aboriginal men, even if assisted with job training and placement (Z = 0), they will still become homeless (Y = 1), due to discrimination in the housing market.

The distinction between conditions (c) and (d) above represents an interaction between race and unemployment in the determination of homelessness, and this sort of interaction is going to cause problems for the interpretation of the controlled direct effect. In this population, the total racial disparity is simply the contrast of the homelessness risk among aboriginal men versus the homelessness risk among white men. Absent any intervention, following conditions (a) and (b) above, men of both races will be made homeless by the crisis, and therefore, the total disparity is $(1 - 1) = 0$. In contrast to the total disparity, the controlled direct effect is the contrast of the homelessness risk among aboriginal men versus the homelessness risk among white men given that a job training and placement intervention makes all men employed, which sets Z from 0 to 1. Following conditions (c) and (d) above, this contrast becomes $(1 - 0) = 1$. Surprisingly, the portion of the racial disparity that is mediated by Z is larger than the overall disparity itself, which upends the whole notion of decomposing or partitioning an observed disparity into its constituent direct and indirect pathways. The idea that the mediator might act differently in the two populations is not at all far-fetched. In fact, social scientists use the term *intersectionality* to refer to the general expectation that all treatments can be expected to be heterogeneous over strata of race, ethnicity, and other axes of identity.[24]

For a real-life example of the decomposition strategy applied to a racial disparity, let's take a paper from the psychology literature, one that sits at the intersection with education and criminology.[25] In a well-cited 2018 paper in the journal *Developmental Psychology*, James Barnes and Ryan Motz considered the overrepresentation of Black Americans in the criminal justice system and proposed that perhaps some portion of this inequality could be attributed to differential exposure to school discipline. There is a large and active literature on this hypothesized "school-to-prison pipeline." The authors advanced this research program with their paper using a large and nationally representative sample, the National Longitudinal Study of Adolescent to Adult Health (Add Health), to estimate the proportion of the overall racial gap that can be attributed to unequal exposure to school-based punishments. The Add Health study sampled students in their middle schools and high schools in the mid-1990s and followed them into adulthood. The authors focused their analyses on about 8,700 students who had identified themselves as either Black or white.

Having been arrested at some point by adulthood was reported by 27.2 percent of the sample, including among seventy-three respondents who were incarcerated at the time of the follow-up interview and completed the interview from prison. The mediator of interest was a history of being

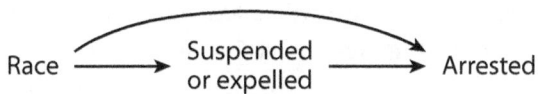

Figure 10.6 Hypothesized relationships between student race, student suspension or expulsion, and later arrest.

expelled or suspended while a student in secondary school, and this was reported by 25.3 percent of the sample. The authors also considered a vast array of measured covariates that might confound these associations, including social, economic, school system, and neighborhood factors. The goal of the causal mediation analysis was to decompose the overall racial disparity in arrest into the portion that was mediated by school discipline and the portion that was not (figure 10.6). This quantity has the causal interpretation that removing the differential application of school discipline would block that indirect pathway and thus eliminate that portion of the arrest disparity. The authors chose natural effects, rather than controlled effects, to better answer the question: What would the disparity look like if there were no differential effect of race on school discipline? This is analogous to giving Black students the school discipline experience of their white peers. Note that the use of natural effects avoids the interaction problem described in the earlier unemployment and housing example, which can invalidate decompositions based on the controlled effects. Moreover, the use of controlled effects would require that all students be disciplined or, alternatively, that no students be disciplined, and neither extreme is a sensible policy objective. A more realistic policy goal is that students would face a disciplinary regime that is not racially biased, which makes the natural effect parameter the more persuasive choice.

The authors found that Black students had more than threefold higher odds of being expelled or suspended, but this was reduced to a 76 percent excess odds after accounting for measured confounders. On the absolute scale, adjusted risk of suspension/expulsion was 15.6 percent for white students and 24.5 percent for Black students.[26] The stark disparity in school discipline between Black and white students, even after adjusting for such a rich set of covariates, speaks to the pervasive racism that must be at play in the typical school environment.

Having established the causal arrow from race to school discipline, the next question is the link between race and arrest, controlling for covariates. Here the authors found an adjusted excess odds of 61 percent, slightly higher than the crude disparity (this is partly a function of the strange behavior of the odds ratio described in chapter 9). The authors then added the school discipline mediator to the regression model and estimated the disparity with the additional adjustment, thus shutting down the mediating pathway. Simply adding the mediator variable to a regression model is a common way of conducting a mediation analysis, as noted earlier, but it is incorrect in this setting. The reason is that many of the covariates that confound the mediator and the outcome are also on indirect paths between race and the outcome. Take poverty, for example, which is carefully measured in the Add Health study and dutifully controlled by the authors. Some portion of the racial disparity in arrest is mediated by the pathway that Black race increases exposure to poverty, which affects both school discipline and arrest (figure 10.7). This is not problematic for the controlled direct effect because variation in the mediator is eliminated by that estimand. For natural effects, however, which are the focus of this analysis, it is prohibited to adjust for any covariate that is affected by the exposure, and surely every social, economic, and neighborhood variable is affected in some way by race. This is why VanderWeele and Robinson insisted that the mediator values for the disadvantaged group must be drawn randomly from the observed distribution of the advantaged group; their proposed statistical method cleverly avoids the pitfall of shutting down additional indirect pathways. Barnes and Motz cited the VanderWeele and Robinson paper but inexplicably did not follow this crucial analytic advice.[27] To be fair, they have a lot of company—it is still rare to find published papers that generate the recommended analysis in this circumstance.[28]

Overlooking the technical error for now, the authors arrived at a natural direct effect estimate of 52.9 percent higher odds of arrest. This finding can be interpreted as the degree to which a racial disparity in arrest would

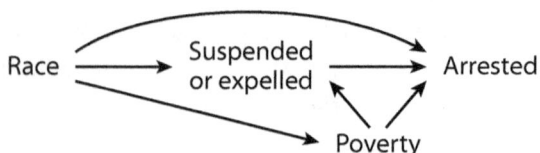

Figure 10.7 Hypothesized relationships between student race, student suspension or expulsion, and later arrest, showing that poverty is a mediator-outcome confounder that is affected by race.

remain even if other covariates were balanced and school discipline were race blind. From the direct and indirect effects, the authors calculated that the proportion mediated was 16.4 percent, implying that the racial disparity in arrests could be reduced by this proportion if schools managed to eliminate racial bias in disciplinary actions.

Considering the context of mass incarceration and the enormous economic and social disruption it entails across our society, this 16 percent reduction in arrests would be highly consequential. It speaks to the insidiously pervasive nature of life-course exposures to racism and the toll that they can take. The numbers are probably not exactly right here, due to the analytic errors and the inherent difficulty in estimating natural effects, but the disparities observed here are large, and one cannot deny the general direction of the results. In response to growing evidence of this school-to-prison pipeline, the federal government had issued a civil rights guidance in 2014 prodding schools to reduce racial and ethnic disparities in disciplinary actions against students. This guidance was rescinded under the first Trump administration in 2018, however, citing work by the criminologist John Paul Wright claiming a genetic basis for the problematic behavior of Black students.[29] Racial inequities in school discipline thus remain rampant to this day.[30]

Mediation remains an essential statistical activity because so much science is devoted to understanding the path-specific mechanisms underlying observed effects. Some of these mechanisms are worked out through experiments, trials, and other interventional designs. Statistical models for mediated effects are also defined and used in published articles across the social sciences. Unfortunately, it is probably not an overstatement to say that most published examples are rather weak. Mediation models are difficult to interpret causally because of demanding measurement, homogeneity, and no-confounding assumptions. Mediated disparity work has proven especially difficult in practice. The VanderWeele and Robinson article in 2014 proposed one principled way forward, so that researchers could estimate the proportion of an observed disparity that would be eliminated if the mediator were to be assigned equitably, without racial preference. Unfortunately, few researchers have attended carefully to their advice, and compelling examples of successful mediation in the disparities context are still rare to come across.

What is perhaps especially useful for us as consumers of published research is to think carefully about what effect is being estimated by a given adjustment. Is the adjusted variable a potential confounder, something that is a common cause of the treatment and the outcome, and therefore, does it bias the effect of the treatment? Or is the adjusted variable a mediator, affected by the treatment and lying on a pathway between the treatment and the outcome? Does it define a mechanism, like a row of falling dominos, by which a treatment reaches the outcome? In that case, the adjustment turns the overall effect into a path-specific effect by blocking one route and leaving the others. It is frustrating that authors, especially in the biomedical sciences, can be very ambiguous about which of these scenarios they have in mind. They tend to adjust for variables that they have available in the dataset simply because they are available, and they view a statistically significant coefficient (see chapter 8) as vindication for that choice. All too often, the interpretation is limited to the fact that the treatment remains "significant," despite the adjustment, and this can be a disastrous strategy because it conflates confounding and mediation, which have diametrically opposed interpretations.[31] One final example helps illustrate this concern.

Writing in the *Journal of Allergy and Clinical Immunology* in 2017, the pediatrician Sharmilee Nyenhuis and colleagues sought to explain racial differences in immune responses among asthmatic children and adults.[32] Asthma is a long-term inflammatory condition of the airways that causes restricted breathing and exhibits a profound racial disparity in the United States.[33] In roughly a thousand asthmatic participants, the authors compared white blood cell counts and defined an eosinophilic response type as one in which this particular type of white blood cell accounted for more than 2 percent of the infiltrating cells. The 264 Black participants had worse profiles on a number of measures of disease severity, including lower forced expiratory volume, higher levels of immunoglobulin E, and a much higher proportion with "uncontrolled" asthma, defined based on frequency of symptoms. About 90 percent of the overall sample were using inhaled corticosteroids, but 95 percent of the Black participants were.

The crude analysis revealed no difference in inflammation profile between the racial groups. The proportions of Black and white patients with an eosinophilic subtype were 19 percent versus 16 percent among those taking corticosteroids, respectively, and 39 percent versus 35 percent among those who were not, respectively, with neither difference being statistically or clinically significant. That could have been the end of the story, but the authors were not satisfied with these real-world proportions and opted instead to adjust for the variables available in the dataset to see what might happen. They don't explain the purpose of this adjustment, the bias that they hope to remove, or even the interpretation of the adjusted disparity, focusing only on whether conditioning on available covariates can make the race p-value smaller (see chapter 8). A logistic regression model was therefore fit conditional on age, sex, and proxy measures of allergic response, adiposity, and lung function. They also adjusted for symptom frequency (controlled versus uncontrolled asthma). The fact of the matter is that the Black participants were sicker in every measure, and by making this adjustment, the authors are implicitly asking: What would the racial disparity be in immunological subtype if the Blacks in the study were *not* sicker but instead balanced with whites on all these factors? Are these covariates meant to be confounders or mediators? The authors do not say. But the adjustment can be imagined conceptually as matching participants on all of these factors, essentially finding a Black and a white subject who are the same age, same adiposity, same lung function, and so on, and then among these matched pairs, calculating the average difference in proportions of the eosinophilic response type. In reality, there are not enough observations to find such matched pairs, but the logistic regression model is meant to approximate the same idea through various linearity and homogeneity assumptions.

Conditional on the covariates, the model estimated that Black participants had 58 percent higher odds of exhibiting eosinophilic airway inflammation among those taking inhaled corticosteroids ($p = 0.046$). The p-value had crossed the magic line, making this a publishable result, and the authors concluded that "African American subjects exhibit greater eosinophilic airway inflammation, which might explain the greater asthma burden in this population."[34] Of course this stated conclusion is not factually correct. In the real world of the crude data, the Black participants in the study had essentially the same proportion of the inflammatory phenotype as whites, and they were sicker. The stated result pertains to what would have been observed, according to the model assumptions, had the Black study subjects somehow not been sicker. Whether this is even a sensible question is surely open for debate. Patients with eosinophilic inflammatory subtype compose just under 20 percent of the asthmatic participants in this sample, and these tend to be the cases most responsive to corticosteroid treatment.[35] Adjusting for "uncontrolled asthma" among a stratum of corticosteroid users is therefore a bit like controlling the final baseball game score for the number of batters on base. Is the covariate a cause of the outcome or a consequence of it? The most sensible interpretation that I can make of this model is that it answers the question of what outcome prevalence would be necessary to balance the disease severity indicators. That is, an eosinophilic inflammatory type is associated with greater responsiveness to corticosteroid treatment, and so to observe Blacks and whites with equal disease severity, it would be necessary for their eosinophilic subtype prevalence to be higher. And voilà—an adjusted odds ratio of 1.58.

If our goal were to mimic a randomized trial, we would indeed want to balance all baseline covariates, that is, the covariates temporally prior to the treatment. But the treatment in this case is Black race, and so nothing in the dataset is temporally prior, nor could the treatment be assigned at random. The fact that the supposed racial difference emerged only in an adjusted model and not in the crude data is omitted completely from the press release and extensive news coverage of the publication.[36] Indeed, the press release extrapolated further, offering that "African Americans may be less responsive to asthma treatment and more likely to die from the condition, in part, because they have a unique type of airway inflammation." And thus an outcome that is reckoned to be 58 percent more common among imaginary Black participants that are somehow less severely affected by asthma is inexplicably transformed into a unique racial trait, something that makes the Black and white subjects sound intrinsically distinct. This elision is outrageous, but of course, it occurs in the press release, which is not subject to peer review.

We have seen that statistical adjustments are central to the task of *explaining* racial and ethnic disparities. This is a difficult task, and we have seen some examples of ways in which it can go awry. Statistical adjustments require structural assumptions, and when the authors do not provide structural rationales for their analytic decisions, the interpretation can be tricky at best. The scientific literature is overflowing with similarly disturbing examples of well-meaning authors applying the tools of quantitative inference too loosely or carelessly and therefore sometimes generating confusion and misunderstanding. Mediation seems like it could be a powerful tool for identifying specific pathways by which disparities emerge, but the success of these techniques is still largely unrealized in practice. For such models to yield valid insights, authors must attend carefully to structural assumptions that are rooted in firm substantive knowledge and statistical assumptions that are testable and subject to empirical refutation. Although we have made a lot of technical progress in the last twenty years, we are not quite there yet.

CHAPTER XI

Nature Versus Nurture

The British National Institute for Healthcare Excellence, which goes by the amiable acronym NICE, recommends that British adults under age fifty-five and without type 2 diabetes who are diagnosed with elevated blood pressure (hypertension) should be first offered a drug called an *angiotensin-converting enzyme (ACE) inhibitor*.[1] This is a long-standing antihypertensive treatment, having been isolated from the venom of Brazilian pit vipers back in the 1950s, and routinely prescribed since the 1970s.[2] The only exception to this standard first-line treatment guideline is for those with "Black African or African–Caribbean family origin," for whom the recommended first-line drug in the United Kingdom is instead a *calcium channel blocker*. The comparable American guideline for treatment of hypertension is the periodic report of the Joint National Committee (JNC), the most recent update of which was the JNC-8 in 2014.[3] These American recommendations are a bit looser, allowing for more classes of drugs to be considered as first-line agents, but like their British counterparts, they also divide the population primarily between Black and non-Black patients.[4] The JNC-8 report does not define anywhere what exactly it means by the terms *Black* and *non-Black*,[5] but they cite as evidence for this treatment distinction the results of a large randomized trial called ALLHAT.[6] In the ALLHAT study, race was defined by self-report as Black, white, Asian, Native American, and other. Although 92 percent of the trial participants identified as white, the latter four categories were combined together and reported in the results as a single non-Black category.

The ALLHAT trial was conducted across more than six hundred clinical sites in the United States, Canada, and the Caribbean from 1994 to 1998. Hypertensive patients were randomized to initiate treatment with one of three classes of drugs: diuretics, ACE inhibitors, or calcium channel blockers. Doctors could switch the patients later if they were not responding adequately or were not tolerating the drugs. This decision was left to the individual clinicians, who of course were not blinded to the patients' racial identities. About 10 percent of the patients were switched from their initial assignments within the first year, and about 20 percent were switched by the end of the trial for two of the drugs. Almost a third of patients had been switched away from the ACE inhibitors by year five. The average systolic blood pressure at the end of the trial was highest in those taking ACE inhibitors by about 2 millimeters of mercury over the group taking diuretics, but this difference was about 4 millimeters of mercury for Black patients, which was the basis for the JNC-8 guideline distinction.[7]

From the discussion of randomization in chapter 2, you may recall that this procedure guarantees that all potential confounders will be balanced between the randomized groups. But keep in mind that patients were randomized to the drugs they received at the start of the trial, not to their race. Therefore, two Black patients who started out with different drugs at the beginning of the trial could be expected to have similar severity of disease and similar social circumstances on average, but this would not be expected of any comparison between Blacks and non-Blacks, who would differ in all the ways that Blacks and non-Blacks differ in society generally, in diet and occupation, material conditions, and so forth. Therefore, even though ALLHAT was a randomized trial, it is important to bear in mind that the race comparison does not benefit in any way from that randomized design. Moreover, the treating physicians maintained control over the dosages delivered and over the switching of patients from one treatment to another, harboring whatever beliefs they might have about the significance of race or other individual patient factors. A significant portion of all patients switched treatments, allowing for selection bias due to beliefs of the physicians, preferences of the patients, or characteristics that were not balanced across race groups, like coexisting health conditions. For example, 12 percent of non-Blacks in the trial had abnormal heart wall thickness at baseline compared to 24 percent of Blacks. There are various clinical interventions to restore blood flow to the heart if it is restricted by arterial plaque, collectively called coronary revascularization, and 17 percent of non-Black patients had received such treatments at the beginning of the ALLHAT trial compared to 5 percent of Blacks. And there were many other baseline differences between the racial groups.

Despite these serious reservations, let's take the ALLHAT results at face value and ask what these results might imply for differential treatment by race. That is, suppose it were true that the expected blood pressure reduction for Black patients was 2 millimeters of mercury or even 4 millimeters of mercury less than for non-Blacks when treated with ACE inhibitors. Would this difference motivate a race-specific treatment plan? It clearly would not. Recall from chapter 7 that a difference in the average response by group does not inform a useful individual response prediction if the spread around each group average is larger than this difference. This is exactly how it looks for blood pressure reduction in response to treatment by ACE inhibitors.[8] A review of about a dozen trials involving hypertensive Black and white participants as of 2007 showed the average white participant lost 10.7 millimeters of mercury and the average Black participant lost 6.8. But 95 percent of the white changes ranged between a rise of 13 and a fall of 34 millimeters, whereas 95 percent of the Black changes ranged between an increase of 22 millimeters and a fall of 35.[9]

Even though the expected response of white patients is larger by almost 4 millimeters, the vast majority of all patients respond similarly, in the sense that they fall under both of the race-specific curves shown in figure 11.1.[10] Such a modest difference between the averages cannot form the basis for a categorical distinction in the treatment strategy when the range of responses is so wide. When a patient walks into the doctor's office, there is no way to know how that individual patient will respond, and you can imagine them being randomly drawn from the distributions depicted in figure 11.1. Suppose the physician needs for the patient's systolic pressure to fall by 10 millimeters. Based on the values shown earlier, 52 percent of white patients will obtain a response at least this big and so will 41 percent of Black patients. Why is this too little an advantage on which to base the treatment algorithm?[11] Suppose the doctor had a hundred white patients and a hundred Black patients and assigned this drug only to the white patients. Then forty-eight of the one hundred white patients (who didn't respond to the drug they got) and forty-one of the one hundred Black patients (who would have responded to the drug they didn't get) were all mistreated by

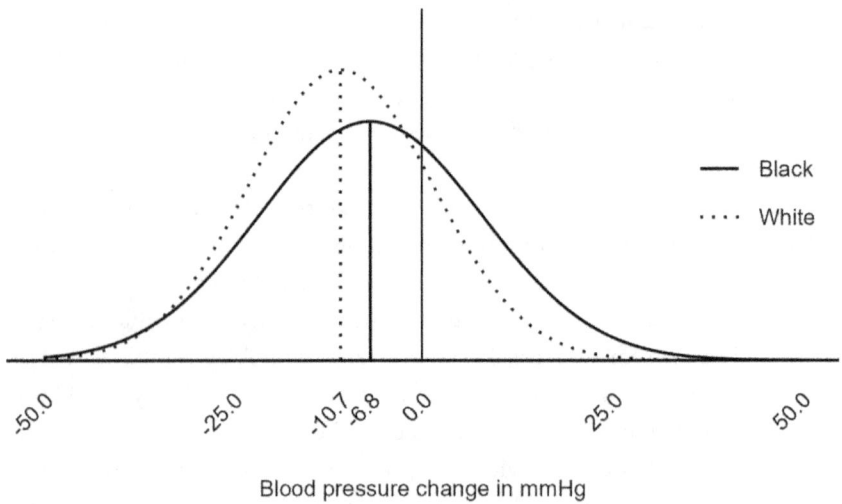

Figure 11.1 Expected change in systolic blood pressure associated with ACE-inhibition therapy, by race.

this treatment algorithm. This is eighty-nine of the two hundred patients, or about 45 percent. It is simply inadmissible to propose a treatment strategy that mistreats almost half of the patients.[12] Of course, race may be better than using no predictor at all because even a tiny amount of information is better than no information.[13] But why must it be a choice of race or nothing? Is there really no other clinical variable that could better segregate the population into responders and nonresponders?[14] How about weight or sex? These might be equally or more important in predicting response to ACE inhibitors, for example,[15] but these variables are not used to distinguish initial treatments in any existing guidelines.[16]

This example raises the broader question: If race does such a poor job of discriminating between responders and nonresponders in this instance, why was it ever included in the guidelines to differentiate treatment strategies? One answer is that hypertension has a particularly long history of being wrapped up with racial myths and hypotheses. In Black Americans, this disease has frequently been described as physiologically distinct and inherently pathological, such as in medical journal articles with titles like "Hypertension in Blacks: Is it a Different Disease?" and "Hypertension in African-Americans: A Paradigm of Metabolic Disarray."[17] It was commonly stated in peer-reviewed articles that Black Americans had the highest blood pressures in the world, even though this was demonstrably false, and European popu-lations with higher average pressures, like Finns, were never described with the same language of innate physiological defect.[18] Because of the reflex-ive elision of race with genetics and therefore the persistent connotation of denoting some sort of human subspecies, the problem of excess Black hypertension was often blithely asserted to have a genetic basis. An endless succession of bizarre theories arose to explain this phenomenon, from wild speculation about the blood pressure effects of skin pigmentation to the all-too-predicable suggestion that it must have something to do with excess testosterone levels in Black men.[19]

One particularly infamous foray into the racial mythology of hyperten-sion was the *slavery hypertension hypothesis*, in which an evolutionary tale was concocted about differential mortality during the Middle Passage from Africa to the New World.[20] The story spun was that high mortality on slave ships was exacerbated by fluid loss from sweating and diarrheal dis-ease, giving a survival advantage to those with the genetic propensity to retain sodium, a trait that would later become lethal in the high-salt diet of modern industrial America. Even some academic luminaries like Jared Diamond endorsed this just-so story,[21] despite an absence of any supporting evidence. When geneticists started to actually accumulate alleles related to blood pressure regulation in the genomic era, however, the scientists found no smoking gun—there were no important risk alleles found to be differ-entially distributed between Blacks in the New World and their ancestral populations in Africa.[22] The theory gradually faded away, despite having wormed its way into all the major hypertension textbooks of the 1990s. It stands as a testament to how eager American medicine was to view excess Black hypertension through the lens of racial essentialism and biological determinism. It also helps to explain why race could be seen as a sufficiently fundamental distinction to be inserted into treatment guidelines—that the disease in this population was considered sui generis and thus in need of its own distinct consideration.

The categorization of humanity into this binary of Black or non-Black is anthropologically absurd and reflects a distinctly American social outlook, forged as it was by its particular history of slavery and Jim Crow. It is true that there are average genetic distances between various populations, just as your brother is more genetically similar to you than your cousin. But at the population level, these are continuous gradations of average related-ness, not categorical distinctions of kind. A Black person randomly sampled from Ethiopia or Kenya may well be more closely related to a white person sampled from Europe or the Middle East than they will be to another Black person from West or southern Africa.[23] There is little biological coherence to these broad racial categories, and so they are not informative about medically or socially relevant traits beyond skin color, if that. Bougainville Islanders, an ethnic group in Papua New Guinea, have among the darkest skin of all humans but are "non-Black" in the sense of having no direct relatedness to sub-Saharan Africans.[24] Nor of course is the light skin of people with albinism considered to confer any racial significance.

The example of skin color is instructive, however, because it demonstrates the adaptation of human beings to local environmental conditions and the more profound point that genetic variations cannot be described as beneficial or harmful in general but only with respect to specific environments. There is still a lot that we don't understand about the origins and mechanisms of human variation in skin color. Our closest primate relatives do not have pigmented skin. It probably emerged over a million years ago concurrently with the loss of hair over most of the human body as a protection against damage from ultraviolet (UV) radiation.[25] Pressure to maintain this trait of darker skin was diminished among those who migrated more recently to higher latitudes, however, because sunlight is less direct and because people in colder climates tend to wear more clothing. Darker skin at higher latitudes might not only be unnecessary but perhaps even deleterious because lighter skin facilitates greater endogenous production of vitamin D. This skin color adaption to life far from our equatorial origins seems to have happened several times in human history, independently in different populations.[26] The complex gradations of skin color observed today also reflect influences of other factors such as altitude, diet, and migration.

The dark pigment in skin is called melanin, and the cells that produce this pigment are called melanocytes. When cancer develops in these cells, it is referred to as melanoma, the most deadly form of skin cancer. The main risk factor for developing melanoma is simply having lighter skin exposed to too much UV radiation, and the highest rates in the world occur among people with lighter skin living close to the equator, especially northern Europeans living in Australia and New Zealand.[27] Now suppose you are an epidemiologist looking for genetic causes of disease using a linear regression model like those discussed in chapter 7. Say the genotype (G) is coded 0 for a person with light skin and coded 1 for a person with dark skin. Now say we also consider two possible environments (E), one in the United Kingdom

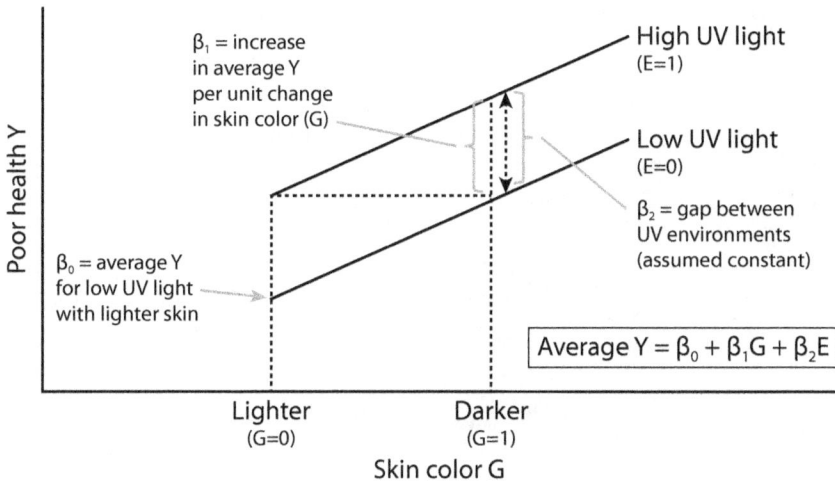

β_1 = increase in average Y per unit change in skin color (G)

High UV light (E=1)

Low UV light (E=0)

β_2 = gap between UV environments (assumed constant)

β_0 = average Y for low UV light with lighter skin

Average $Y = \beta_0 + \beta_1 G + \beta_2 E$

Lighter (G=0)

Darker (G=1)

Skin color G

Poor health Y

Figure 11.2 Schematic representation of the relationship between skin color and UV radiation exposure using a linear regression model with no interaction term.

with low UV radiation coded 0 and one in northern Australia with high UV radiation, coded 1. As we did previously in chapter 7, the researcher might naively set this up as a linear regression model with slope parameters for the G and E effects on overall health (Y) (figure 11.2).

Mathematics cares nothing about reality, and so any statistical software program is happy to fit this model and provide predictions, but this model is horrifically wrong and its predictions will be garbage. Because the terms enter additively, the two lines are parallel, with a constant gap between them. This model specification therefore assumes that the effect of genotype (β_1) is constant across environments and that the effect of environments (β_2) is constant across genotypes. The model assumption of effect constancy that is made here is completely false because dark skin (G = 1) is advantageous in a high UV light environment (E = 1) where it prevents melanoma but disadvantageous in a low UV light environment (E = 0) where it impedes production of vitamin D. Likewise, light skin (G = 0) is disadvantageous in a high UV light environment (E = 1) but advantageous in a low UV light environment (E = 0) by the same logic. This means that the two lines cannot be parallel, and in fact, one must be sloping up and the other must be sloping down. To allow this to happen, we need to add another parameter in the model, which is the interaction of genes and environments and which is

Average $Y = \beta_0 + \beta_1 G + \beta_2 E + \beta_3 GE$

β_1 = increase in average Y per unit change in skin color (G) with low UV light (E=0)

β_2 = gap between UV environments with lighter skin

Low UV light (E=0)

High UV light (E=1)

β_0 = average Y for low UV light with lighter skin

Poor health Y

Lighter (G=0)

Darker (G=1)

Skin color G

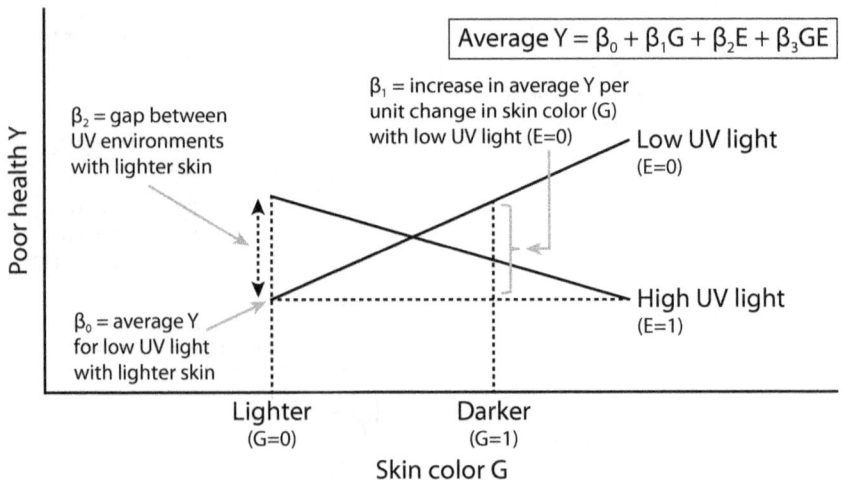

Figure 11.3 Schematic representation of the relationship between skin color and UV radiation exposure using a linear regression model with a product interaction term.

modeled as the multiplication of E × G.[28] The new regression model then looks like the one shown in figure 11.3.

The additional product interaction term allows for there to be an increasing slope of poor health with darker skin in low UV light ($\beta_1 > 0$), whereas there is a decreasing slope of poor health with darker skin in high UV light [$(\beta_1 + \beta_3) < 0$].[29] This model specification is able to capture the key logic of local adaptation, which is that a trait is not beneficial or harmful in any absolute sense but only in the context of a specific environment. There are some traits that are good for everyone always, and these tend not to vary across populations, like the genes that tell our bodies to grow a pancreas. But where there are traits that do vary between populations, especially recent adaptations like light skin or the sickling of red blood cells to combat infection by malaria, these generally arise because they are beneficial in specific environments and irrelevant or perhaps harmful in others.[30] The reason to focus on this point in a book about statistical analysis of racial and ethnic disparities is to raise suspicion of the common tendency to offer genetic explanations for these disparities, especially based on statistical adjustments for concomitant social and environmental factors. As shown earlier, when gene × environment interactions are contemplated, the effects of the genetic variants are not isolated by such adjustments but rather can only be interpreted in stratifications of those conditions.

Consider the concept of *heritability*, a frequently used term in the genetics literature that is most often interpreted as the proportion of variation in a trait that is due to genes rather than environments.[31] For example, based on studies of twins (comparing identical twins who share 100 percent of alleles with fraternal twins who share only 50 percent), intelligence is often asserted to have a heritability of about 50 percent, implying equal contributions of genes and environments. In fact, there is something of a longstanding crisis in human genetics regarding the fact that we do not find variants that account for much of this supposed genetic causation, a problem referred to as the *missing heritability problem*.[32] But this apparent crisis is simply a consequence of heritability being an absurd notion in the first place because there can be no general statement of what percentage of observed variation is a result of genes without reference to environments.[33]

Take the simple example offered by the epidemiologist Ken Rothman of phenylketonuria, a disease in which a person with a rare genetic variant (the PKU allele) cannot metabolize an amino acid called phenylalanine if it is encountered in the diet.[34] If you have the PKU allele and you are exposed to dietary phenylalanine, severe intellectual disability results. So what percentage of this effect is genetic? One hundred percent of the cases of cognitive damage from phenylketonuria would be prevented if the affected person did not have the PKU allele, so in that sense, the disease is 100 percent genetic. But 100 percent of the cases of cognitive damage from phenylketonuria would also be prevented if the affected person were not exposed to dietary phenylalanine, and in that sense, the disease is also 100 percent environmental. In sum, the notion of a single number for the "heritability" of a trait is completely bogus. Some geneticists have pointed out that the supposed missing heritability problem can be explained entirely by such interactions, but somehow the simplistic concept of heritability persists.[35] Now imagine two racial or ethnic groups with equal frequencies of the PKU allele but with different exposures to dietary phenylalanine. The group with the higher dietary exposure would have greater incidence of a "genetic" disease, even when there is no genetic difference between the groups at all.

It's meaningless to discuss the effects of genes without reference to environments, in the same way that you can't discuss the ideal choice of clothing without making any reference to the weather. Is the snowsuit or the bikini the better general attire in some abstract sense? And yet researchers do often refer to isolating genetic effects in exactly this way. Take one example by Erik Corona and colleagues, who calculated the independent genetic risk of more than one hundred diseases across more than fifty populations and reported that the genetic propensity for type 2 diabetes was highest in Africa and declined as populations migrated out of Africa, reaching its lowest levels in aboriginal populations of the Pacific and the New World.[36] "Ethnic background plays a surprisingly large role in how diabetes develops on a cellular level," announced the accompanying press release from Stanford University.[37] The inconvenient problem with this proposed geographic pattern of genetic risk, however, is that it is the opposite of what is actually observed in the real world, where Africans have relatively low levels of diabetes, whereas Asian and New World populations experience higher levels. After their paper was published, I posted a comment online at the journal website pointing out this obvious anomaly.[38] The authors responded swiftly and perhaps indignantly: "The primary objection you raise to this research is based on a common misconception that observed risk and genetic risk of complex disease are expected to agree."[39]

The authors have a point, and of course the reason these estimates won't necessarily agree is because disease is *mostly* a function of environment, which the authors have pointedly excluded from consideration. The authors therefore treat "genetic risk" as a latent (unobserved) potential that would be hypothetically observed only if there were no environment of any kind. This is not like a person with the PKU allele in a world with no dietary phenylalanine because "no dietary phenylalanine" is itself an environment. Rather, the genetic risk in this framework operates in some kind of more abstract world in which diets don't even exist; only genes exist. The authors further reinforced the point that the target quantity is completely metaphysical: "[Estimating the genetic risk] requires neither empirical evidence about disease occurrence nor other methodology grounded in epidemiology. Inclusion of such data would be gratuitous and unnecessary to address the stated question." Thus, the genetic risks of disease reported in the paper are not only independent of data on disease in the real world but also can never be refuted by any such data. This is reminiscent of the ancestry proportions discussed in chapter 6, which can never be shown to be incorrect because they can never be contradicted by evidence. Once again, this raises nagging philosophical questions like the old demarcation problem about what separates science from metaphysics and what it means to study things that can never be manifested in the observable world.[40] If nobody can ever experience this latent genetic risk, why would anyone care about it?

Here is another thought experiment to complicate the strict nature versus nurture duality, offered by the sociologist Christopher Jencks more than fifty years ago.[41] Imagine a society in which there is discrimination against children with red hair. These redheads are therefore exposed to various deprivations; they are given inadequate nutrition and are denied access to good schools. As a result, there is an observed correlation between the trait of red hair and low educational attainment, low measured IQ, and so on. This correlation does not arise from confounding, however, in the sense that genetic manipulation of the red hair alleles in an embryo to change the hair color of the child would actually prevent this deprivation given the prevailing social environment in which the child would be raised. Thus, a genetic variant responsible for red hair is a true cause of low educational attainment and low IQ in this social context. In contrast, an example of confounding is that in early twentieth-century America, tuberculosis was so common among Irish immigrants that scientists proposed that unknown genetic factors responsible for tuberculosis must be linked to the genes that caused red hair.[42] Unlike the Jencks example, this is spurious—Irish immigrants were poor, and poverty was a cause of tuberculosis infection because it was linked to crowding and poor nutrition. You can tell it's confounded and not causal because you know that if you changed their hair color, it would not change their risk of tuberculosis.

Because the Jencks example is truly causal, not spurious, it challenges the categorical distinction between genetic and environmental explanations for disparities as logically meaningful. With respect to variation in some trait, "nature" and "nurture" are simply not two distinct bins of variation that can be summed to obtain the total variation. Rather, as in Jencks's case, sometimes one works through the other. Or consider this example. Suppose that a parent has a genetic propensity to create an orderly and intellectually stimulating home for their child and that this environment causes the child to have higher educational attainment and higher IQ. This is a truly causal genetic effect mediated by the environment.[43] Similarly, through the mechanism of social influences on mate choice, there are many environmental effects mediated by genetics.[44] We can't say there are two distinct bins labeled "nature" and "nurture." Instead, there's an intricate web of causation, with myriad strands that cross, fuse, and interconnect. The era of simplistic, Manichean genetics is behind us.

Claims of genetic causation for observed racial and ethnic disparities are ubiquitous in the scientific literature. This is especially true in biomedicine, where medical researchers have long posited "biological" explanations for almost every imaginable health condition where a racial difference is observed. This seems to often lean in one direction, however, in the sense that when there is an excess of disease in white people, it tends not be to so essentialized.[45] Take the example of cancer. In the early part of the twentieth century, it appeared to medical professionals that cancer was primarily a disease of white women, and therefore, it was seen more as an affliction of excess refinement and culture.[46] When Black men were found to have much higher prostate cancer incidence and mortality, however, the prevailing cultural associations of Black male sexuality cast the surfeit as an inherent defect of excess testosterone.[47] Indeed, if you just think of any prevailing racial stereotype, you can bet that there is a paper somewhere claiming to justify that stereotype with the discovery of some genetic variant. For instance, a 2005 paper in the journal *Science* claimed to have found a novel mutation arising about six thousand years ago that made European brains larger than those of Africans.[48] The authors speculated that this novel mutation could have accounted for the European inventions of agriculture and written language (things that Europeans did not actually invent).[49] Needless to say, this finding did not hold up. And this kind of motivated thinking is not limited to biomedicine. Some eager criminologists have also claimed to find the genetic variants that make adolescents more likely to join a gang,[50] or make Hispanics more likely to become involved with the criminal justice system.[51] There are economists who have proposed a genetic explanation for why Africa is poorer than Europe.[52] And scores of psychologists have spent the last hundred years vigorously arguing that certain races (i.e., the races of those psychologists) are genetically endowed to be more intelligent than other races.[53]

Thus, all branches of social and biomedical science have been touched by the pernicious essentialization of racial categories and have trucked in genetic explanations for observed racial and ethnic disparities. These explanations almost always involve trying to control for the social and material environment in some way to isolate the "independent" contribution of genes—a task that is fundamentally misguided, as we have seen. Even setting aside the issue of interactions, the premise of measurement and adjustment for all environmental factors that affect health, IQ, or behavior is patently absurd. This supposed statistical control was exactly the foundation of the argument in Richard Herrnstein and Charles Murray's 1994 book *The Bell Curve*, which was perhaps the most influential work of racial essentialism in the modern era.[54] Yet the statistical methodology in the book was excoriated by technical experts as wholly inadequate to support the stated conclusion of innate Black cognitive inferiority. "It would be miraculous if fifteen to twenty-three years of environmental influences could be summarized by a composite of education, occupation, and family income measured in one year," scolded James Heckman, the Nobel laureate economist. Heckman's 1995 review pummeled the book on multiple grounds, but in this quote, he was addressing the abject failure to statistically equalize the differences in material and social life experienced by Blacks and whites in twentieth-century America.[55] Environment is a near infinitely large set of conditions, of course, many of which will affect intellectual ability in one way or another. Herrnstein and Murray did not adjust for quality of diet or exposure to lead, for example, or any of the psychological impacts of segregation, or a million other things. How was such an incomplete statistical model ever taken seriously? And yet the book sold more than half a million copies in hardcover.[56] Clearly there was a hunger for this argument—an eagerness to explain away racial disparities as inevitable and immutable.

Simplistic genetic explanations for racial and ethnic disparities may have low scientific credibility for all the reasons outlined earlier, but they loom very large in the popular imagination. Some of the blame for this widespread endorsement of racial essentialism rests with the media, which tend to hype new "findings" but give little attention to assumptions and caveats and even less attention when new claims cannot be replicated and are quietly forgotten. The daily headlines are that some genetic variant is discovered that explains a racial disparity, but there are no headlines when most such claims turn out to be false alarms.[57] In a final example, I recount one such story, in which a dubious message of genetic explanation was promoted uncritically.

In 2011, the geneticist Dara Torgerson and colleagues published a paper in *Nature Genetics* that pooled several epidemiological studies of asthma into a single analysis, which scientists refer to as a *meta-analysis*.[58] The pooled dataset included more than five thousand individuals with various ancestries, and the authors reported a number of variants that were associated with asthma, most of which were consistent across all of the ethnic subpopulations in the dataset. One of the alleles that was found to be associated with asthma had not been previously identified, and the authors reported that it showed variation only in individuals of African descent.[59] The new polymorphism that was observed by these authors to be strongly associated with asthma was located near a gene called PYHIN1 on chromosome 1. The specific DNA nucleotide at that location varied among those with African ancestry but not among those with European ancestry. The authors focused on this as an intriguing finding because of the substantial racial disparity in asthma prevalence in the United States, which occurs in 7.7 percent of white Americans and 12.5 percent of Black Americans.

Could this particular genetic variation in people of African ancestry really be a partial explanation for their excess risk of asthma? Buried deep in an electronic supplement to the paper were the details of the data analysis, however, and it is only in this appendix material where one can discern that in fact the nucleotide present for all people of European descent is the *high* risk variant, meaning that all white people have the form of the gene associated with more asthma, not less asthma. If the variation seen only in Blacks is taken to be a cause of asthma, therefore, the genetic pattern is the opposite of the disease risk that is observed in the population, where whites are observed to have lower risk. Thus, the news coverage of the publication was somewhat surprising: "US researchers have discovered a genetic mutation unique to African Americans that could help explain why Blacks are so susceptible to asthma."[60]

What the authors observed was that being a case of asthma was associated with the nucleotide found at this location in Blacks; no association in whites could be estimated because of the lack of variation. Because DNA is inherited in chunks, variants that are physically proximate on the genome are inherited together, and so from this observed association, one can only conclude that a genetic cause of asthma might be somewhere in the vicinity of this single nucleotide polymorphism (SNP). Nonetheless, the news coverage portrayed this location as if it were the cause of asthma itself: "Because the study was so large and ethnically diverse . . . it enabled the researchers to find this new gene variant that exists only in African Americans and African Caribbeans. This new variant, located in a gene called PYHIN1, is part of a family of genes linked with the body's response to viral infections, [Carole] Ober said. 'We were very excited when we realized it doesn't exist in Europe,'" Ober added.[61]

Why be excited about the lack of variation at this one spot in the population of European ancestry? Everyone has some nucleotide there. It's only that at this particular location, the Black participants have two versions, one of which is associated with less asthma. This version associated with less asthma is the one that the white people don't have. Moreover, the observed association only suggests that a genetic cause of asthma should be somewhere in the same genomic neighborhood as this SNP, so the fact that this particular location has no variation in whites is irrelevant. Even if the investigators got very lucky and this SNP happened to be the actual causal variant, it can't possibly explain higher asthma risk in Blacks because some of them, unlike whites, have a *low-risk* variant at that spot. So no matter how one interprets the study's findings, the news coverage can't be right.

Thinking that this was an example of the press being irresponsibly sensationalistic, I sent a letter to the Reuters science reporter and editor with a copy to the corresponding author from the University of Chicago. The Reuters editor checked with the authors, who responded that they endorsed the news coverage and saw no problem whatsoever. So I wrote to the authors directly, and they were polite but basically said that they didn't want to waste time discussing it with me. They mentioned a few general issues that I should consider, such as interaction, and then they asked to be left alone. Of course potential interactions (discussed earlier in this chapter) are always plausible, but how does this justify describing the result of this paper as an explanation for excess asthma in Black Americans? Sure, it is possible for a risk factor to operate in different directions across two populations, but this is a red herring because there was no mention of any such interaction in the paper. The news reporting connected the paper to a problem of public interest that the authors perhaps thought made a good hook but that did not actually reflect the content of the peer-reviewed article. There could be no evidence of effect heterogeneity across race groups for this variant because there was no effect estimated among whites at all. The authors seemed to view the media interview as an opportunity for connecting their research program to racial disparities, even if no finding in the paper really supported that.

Most of the other examples in this book are chosen from the published literature of the last few years, but this example is from 2011. I chose a sensational claim from more than a decade ago exactly so that we could look to see what came of this much-heralded discovery. As best I can see searching publications for PYHIN1 and racial disparities in asthma since 2011, the SNP that they were so excited about has never again been mentioned in the scientific literature, except in relation to the 2011 paper, and the PYHIN1 gene was not associated with asthma in subsequent studies.[62] There is a widespread phenomenon called *publication bias* in which negative results are rarely reported because journals want exciting, new, headline-producing findings, not disappointing nonfindings.[63] A review of genetic explanations for asthma disparities published in 2019 describes the 2011 result as never being successfully replicated, but this failure to hold up in subsequent studies did not generate any headlines.[64] So the public is left with the memory of the 2011 headline trumpeting a genetic explanation for the observed racial disparity, along with a steady barrage of other such findings, each further reinforcing an essentialist view of racial differences. It's no wonder that people get confused.[65]

Conclusion

Race and ethnicity are social facts in our world, and so we must contend with them. There are certainly those who advocate that these categorizations are outdated and we should move past them. As citizens of multiracial democracies like the United States become more ethnically and culturally mixed over time, the existing delineations may indeed become less salient.[1] But for now, these classifications remain powerful predictors of almost every aspect of life—of educational attainment, of partner selection, of health and disease, of where people live and work, and of their behaviors, affiliations, and political activities. Of course, there is diversity within every defined group and no tendency applies strictly to all members of a category, but important differences persist at the group level. Where groups face differential treatment, we have a societal obligation to monitor inequalities and seek policies to reduce or eliminate them. There are political disagreements about the policy regime for defining and monitoring group differences and especially strong disagreements about potential interventions to achieve some greater sense of "fairness"—a concept that is, on the one hand, simple to understand and, on the other hand, difficult to define formally.[2]

This book accepts the premise that societies have a commitment to observing and recording racial and ethnic identities and to monitoring the distribution of outcomes across these groups in the pursuit of equity. For those who think this whole premise is misguided and does more harm than good, the critique offered here may be moot.[3] But for those who think that racial and ethnic disparities are a legitimate concern, then a central challenge is this: How should these disparities be defined, measured, and interpreted? I hope that the preceding chapters have at the very least demonstrated that these are not trivial questions. It is not obvious what the groups should be, and for many people, it is not obvious how to assign membership to whatever groups are established. Even if we get past these basic measurement issues, it is not easy to define exactly what we want to know about the differences in outcomes between groups and how we should best go about generating, reporting, and interpreting those statistics. There are a lot of problems with how we generally do this now, as I hope I have demonstrated. We can do better. Some of the objectively poor practices described in earlier chapters should simply be abandoned. Even so, navigating these choices depends to some extent on values upon which we are not likely to all agree. To some extent, therefore, monitoring racial and ethnic disparities must remain a political process in which different factions must lobby for their priorities and preferences against the wishes of other factions.

An example of this latter point is the controversy over the potential introduction of a multiracial category in the U.S. census to better accommodate people whose parents are racially discordant. The U.S. Census Bureau has meandered around this issue for much of its history, having included a "mulatto" category in seven censuses between 1850 and 1920 and offering "octoroon" and "quadroon" categories in 1890. The "mulatto" category allowed for "any perceptible trace of African blood," as discerned by the census takers.[4] By the 1960s, census takers were instructed to categorize mixed-race children according to the father's race, while also allowing for some subjective exceptions. Then in 1970, respondents began to select their own race and were instructed to select the one single category that most closely matched their identity. In 1980 and 1990, any respondent who checked more than one race box was reclassified into a single box, until 2000 when respondents were instructed that they could mark as many boxes as they wished. Less than 3 percent of Americans selected multiple races that year, but as the number of mixed marriages increased as well as the social acceptance of complex racial identities, this proportion increased dramatically. There are also important cohort effects, such that a third of those under eighteen had more than one race by the 2020 census compared to only 9 percent of respondents sixty-five years and older.[5] The political debate over the reintroduction of a "multiracial" category revolved around the potential dilution of political and social influence that might result from splitting off the multiracial respondents from their traditional racial group blocks.[6] By allowing respondents to instead check multiple boxes, these totals can still be mobilized as evidence of political power without siphoning off some fraction into a single multiracial box. There is nothing objectively wrong with this way of counting, but the point is that the data collection regime reflects political considerations above and beyond any justification in sociology, history, or biology.

After the groups are defined and we begin to construct disparity measures, then once again the process requires lots of choices. The unambiguous depiction of racial disparity in the real world is the crude contrast, formed as either a difference or a ratio of two statistics. For example, in 2021, there were a little more than a half million births among non-Hispanic Black women in the United States, and 362 of those mothers died in or around pregnancy. We have already discussed ambiguity in who counts as "non-Hispanic Black," and indeed, this number includes only those who indicated a single racial identity. There is also some ambiguity around what constitutes a pregnancy-related death.[7] But accepting these two numbers, the rate is 69.9 maternal deaths per 100,000 live births per year. The comparable numbers for non-Hispanic white women are 503 deaths out of 1,887,656 births, for a rate of 26.6 per 100,000.[8] The disparity can therefore be expressed as a difference of 43.3 deaths per 100,000 births or as a unitless ratio of 2.63. In principle, one could also show the racial contrast for those who survive pregnancy as $\left(\left(\frac{517,537}{517,899}\right) / \left(\frac{1,887,153}{1,887,656}\right)\right) = 0.9996$, which looks very different (although the survival difference measure maintains the same magnitude as the mortality difference). This already presents many options, and we have not yet even age-adjusted or accounted for other imbalances between the groups. In practice, almost all routine reporting focuses on the crude rate ratio of 2.63, which has many limitations, including obscuring the number of excess deaths, as detailed in chapter 9.

Then come additional considerations. Maternal mortality increases dramatically with age; the rate is 20.4 per 100,000 live births for mothers under the age of twenty-five and almost seven times higher (138.5 per 100,000) for mothers who are forty years old or older. White women are older when giving birth: 28.1 years on average at first birth, compared to 25.5 years for Black women in 2021.[9] Is it "fair" to report the crude comparison, which reflects in part the contrast of maternal ages as well as the different social environment by race? As we have seen, this question can only be answered in the context of a set of values and priorities over which we may not all agree. There can be no objective solution to this question, nor is there one solution that is fit for all purposes.

Deciding to account for age—so that we compare Black and white women of the same ages rather than across contrasting ages—may resolve some concerns. But it might raise others. It may force us to grapple with the question of why these population groups have very different fertility patterns by age in the first place and how such patterns differ by state or social class or other potential stratifications. After all, the crude contrast is a fact in the real world, and the adjusted one turns that real contrast into something completely hypothetical. Once we leave reality for imaginary scenarios, how far should we go? If we decide to adjust for age and perhaps other covariates as well, there are choices to be made in how this should be done. Is the increase in mortality risk with age the same for Black and white women, or is that also confounded by social class and general health status? If older Black women are sicker on average, is this also something that should be adjusted away like age? *How* to make these adjustments is a statistical matter. But *whether* to make them is an ethical one.

Randomized trials offer complete causal isolation of the treatment, in the sense that it will not be correlated with any other factor, whether measured or unmeasured. Racial and ethnic disparities can never achieve any similar level of causal isolation, and in fact, the groups must be profoundly unequal on a huge range of other factors simply because race and ethnicity are such powerful forces in our society. Our race influences many things in our lives, from our social affiliation to our life chances to the nature of our interactions with individuals and institutions. It is perhaps an overstatement to say that all such interactions are tainted by racism, but they are at least all tainted by racial awareness. As such, the question of covariate adjustment becomes a potential morass. What does one adjust for? And how does one know when to stop adjusting? It is possible, indeed appropriate, for different investigators to make different decisions about the adjustments to be made. Principled schema have been proposed in specific situations,[10] but the vast majority of reported disparity statistics follow no articulated logic or coherent justification. This is why the landscape of disparities reporting and analysis has become so confused by ad hoc decisions and clouded inferences.

On top of this adjustment dilemma is the even knottier problem of stratified inference discussed in chapter 5, in which restrictions in the study design or the analysis can warp disparities in unexpected directions. We have examined typical situations in which investigators misinterpret these conditional associations, journal reviewers and editors are not generally attentive to these more subtle statistical phenomena, and the news media further obfuscate and sensationalize the results. The quagmire of conditioning on factors downstream from the treatment variable has haunted statistics for decades.[11] The problem of adjusted racial and ethnic disparities is that just about all potential adjustment and stratification factors are downstream of these indicators. In situations where a stratification flips the direction of the disparity, there are two conflicting stories that could be told. It becomes the obligation of the author to motivate either the crude or the conditional estimate as the more salient to report and to offer a justification that accounts for the causal structure of the problem and the specific question that the analysis aims to answer. But this level of accountability is rare in practice.

The large number of choices available to the analyst inevitably creates a garden of forking paths, to use a phrase popularized by the statistician Andrew Gelman.[12] These forking paths give the author a tremendous amount of latitude to select the final result for publication, chosen from among a wide range of potential values that result from different contrast measures, adjustments and stratifications, and model specifications. There's an old trope that statistics is just a clever way to lie with data,[13] but I am not so cynical. I'd rather believe that most people producing quantitative studies of racial and ethnic disparities are sincere and fundamentally honest. But even so, it is inevitable when faced with a range of potential ways of representing the world that we lean, consciously or unconsciously, toward the ones that "look right." The most oft-cited quote in all of statistics is George Box's aphorism that "all models are wrong, but some models are useful."[14] When there are so many choices available to the analysts and so little expectation that these choices be explained or justified, it is natural to begin to wonder: Useful in what way? Useful to whom?

The discussion above concerns surveillance, but as we have seen, the statistical application of racial and ethnic identities goes far beyond mere description, extending also to prediction and explanation. In these realms, the scorecard looks decidedly less benign. Race and ethnicity are frequently included in models predicting a person's outcomes in the economic sphere, in the criminal justice system, and in their health because these variables are highly informative in the aggregate, even if their individual-level prediction is often exceedingly weak. When predictions are adjusted for race, as in the recently abandoned equations for estimating kidney function, they are often poorly justified, don't transport well to other societies, and end up disadvantaging minority individuals.[15] When etiological models of racial disparities are constructed, the results are difficult to interpret and can function to reinforce essentialist mythologies. We saw that experiments and observational designs around differential treatment were viable and often informative but that an explanation rooted in the body of a study subject, rather than in the mind of a decision-maker, was rarely tenable. Especially for environmentally sensitive and behaviorally complex traits like criminality and IQ, explaining racial differences statistically is crippled not only by a lack of causal identification, due to myriad unmeasured common causes, but also by wholly inadequate measures across all elements of the model, rendering the whole effort a dangerous waste of time and resources. Rather than the old computing acronym GIGO for "garbage in, garbage out," these analyses amount to SISO—"stereotypes in, stereotypes out." This is not to say that some scientific questions are too socially delicate to be asked. Rather, it is to say that some scientific questions are too ill-conceived and too poorly specified to be answered.

Where do we go from here? There is no simple fix for such a longstanding and complex web of bad habits, misunderstandings, and perverse incentives, but I can offer some broad points for bending toward progress rather than away from it. First and perhaps most controversially, I think that the preceding litany of statistical failures speaks to the need to decenter race and ethnicity in quantitative functions of government and social science research. I fully appreciate that these designations are sociologically important, but there is no reason to treat them as the central organizing frame for society in every instance. A criminal suspect and a medical patient are regularly identified by age, sex, and race, as though these are always the three most important things you ever need to know about a person. Must these unstable, fuzzy, and atavistic categorizations forever be the dominating guardrails through which we navigate our entire lives? For a medical patient, perhaps the thing you'd rather know right off the bat is their diabetes status or their weight. For the criminal suspect, maybe the more salient trait would be their educational attainment or prior arrest record. In every situation in which we reflexively forefront race and ethnicity, it is worth at least asking if we are perpetuating the dominance of these classifications more than is warranted. Yes, monitoring racial and ethnic inequalities remains a legitimate and important function of government and academia, but this does not mean that racial identity must be displayed prominently like a *Judenstern* in every official interaction and report. Race and ethnicity matter, and this is highlighted with particular clarity through the lens of modern identity politics.[16] But race and ethnicity are not the only important aspects of identity. People also have spirituality, musical tastes, sexuality, political affiliations, regional loyalties, devotions to sports teams, and so many other dimensions to make the human experience infinitely deep and nuanced. A statistical model is already necessarily too simplistic, and one that is premised on a few racial or ethnic labels even more so. We can do better by simply not being so reflexively committed to this one, old, tired set of bins.[17]

On the issue of adjustments, at the very least, we should encourage the routine provision of both crude and adjusted results because this gives the reader a sense of how big of an impact the model exerted. Adjustments should be well-motivated, computer code should be provided, and when appendix pages are available, alternate model specifications can be explored in sensitivity analyses.[18] To achieve more profound changes to practice, however, we probably need to update how statistics is taught for those who are headed toward applied fields, with less emphasis on mathematical formalisms and more on the real-world interpretations of statistics based on observational data. Tests and procedures that are justified under randomization assumptions are less relevant for nonexperimental data, and these can be fruitfully deemphasized in favor of more attention toward sensitivity analyses that investigate the uncertainty associated with the inevitable unmeasured confounders and the selection and measurement errors.[19] In short, we should stop modeling under the ideal conditions that exist only in statistics textbooks and start modeling under the more realistic scenarios in which data live in the wild. Revamped statistical training could also move people away from testing and toward estimation, with an emphasis on confidence interval width as a relative measure of precision.[20] Apparent variation in outcomes across racial and ethnic groups should not be overinterpreted when some strata are small and therefore subject to considerable sampling variability. Indeed, shrinkage (chapter 7) can be very helpful in providing estimates that are more reliable as predictors of true population differences.[21] Most importantly, we must teach applied statistics with greater attention to the substantive considerations that underlie coherent adjustment decisions, such as the values behind distinguishing allowable from nonallowable covariates in disparities studies.[22]

When it comes to explaining racial and ethnic disparities based on observed covariates, it is probably time to move away from the vague abstractions of routine regression adjustments. It is difficult to articulate the assumptions that would give these models causal interpretations and even harder to connect the model estimates to concrete social policies that might be envisioned to narrow the racial gaps. Rather, we should prefer a more overtly causal modeling strategy in which the following question is posed: How will the observed racial disparity change under some specific intervention policy? For example, the epidemiologist Paloma Rojas-Saunero and colleagues recently addressed the question of how existing racial disparities in dementia incidence would be changed if everyone's blood pressures were controlled to normotensive levels.[23] This is a meaningful question because we have routine pharmaceutical interventions to achieve this goal, and we know full well that racial and ethnic groups are currently disparate in their levels of hypertension treatment and control.[24] An interesting dilemma for this modeling exercise is how to handle mortality because blood pressure control allows people to live longer and living longer increases the opportunity to get dementia. This is an unavoidable complication, but the point is that the hypothetical intervention is concrete and feasible, and we have follow-up data on people who are exposed to such interventions to calibrate these predictions accurately.[25] This contrasts with controlling statistically for vague proxies like socioeconomic status indicators, where there is no plausible intervention in view that could equalize such factors. Statistical results come closest to informing real policy decisions when the modeling targets specifically defined laws and programs, such as studies that estimate the racial and ethnic equity impacts of the 2014 Medicaid expansion.[26] A statistics that focuses on predicting the impacts of well-defined interventions is much more potentially informative for real-world decision-making than one that trucks in abstract mathematical constructions like "statistical significance" and "percent of variance explained."[27]

Finally, there are the ethical responsibilities of the analysts. Surely there are some who are intent, consciously or unconsciously, on exaggerating or minimizing racial and ethnic disparities for ideological or careerist motivations, just as there are complex cognitive biases in all quantitative research.[28] Describing and explaining racial and ethnic disparity is an inherently political activity, and so objectivity is not something that we can realistically expect. At the same time, objectivity is something that we can sincerely and relentlessly strive toward. Most people who gravitate to these research questions do so exactly because they care about them in some deep way, and so it is natural that these motivated scientists will exercise statistical judgements that are consistent with their philosophies and ethical priorities.[29] Even so, we can nurture a professional environment that facilitates the convergence of diverse viewpoints into a consensus scientific literature that is pruned of at least the most dissonant of researchers' prior convictions. Openness and transparency with respect to research methodologies, sharing of data, a spirit of constructive peer review, and a willingness to debate and improve, these are the hallmarks of healthy quantitative discourse.

We should accept that graphical and statistical representations of racial and ethnic disparities are not generally right or wrong in any absolute sense but more often better or worse in foregrounding one aspect over another. These choices can almost always benefit from being continuously refined or at least further explored. All quantitative professionals have an obligation to participate actively and constructively in peer review, to improve the overall quality of published work, and to raise expectations for research practice and nuanced interpretation of study results. I have presented and explained dozens of examples of poor practice in the preceding chapters and offered many suggestions for how we can make this science more robust, honest, and useful. It is up to us, as a community of professionals, to enact these improvements and enforce higher expectations for thoughtful representation and interpretation of these data. Unfortunately, we suffer presently from a tragedy of the commons, in which the pressures of a brutally publish-or-perish world incentivize many analysts to cut corners and act selfishly in ways that pollute our accumulating pool of knowledge. This slows progress toward evidenced-based policy innovations that could reduce existing disparities. Nobody can raise the bar for us except ourselves.

Striving toward objectivity in statistical representations of racial and ethnic disparity is not a condemnation of advocacy. The subject matter is inherently political, and people enter into this arena of work exactly because they are driven by profoundly humanistic motivations. At the same time, advocates also need evidence at their disposal to advocate effectively. The statistical management, representation, and modeling of disparities aspire to serve this crucial role, providing the best and most robust evidentiary basis for progress toward a just and humane society, however people envision that goal.

Notes

Acknowledgments

1. Jay S. Kaufman and Richard S. Cooper, "In Search of the Hypothesis," *Public Health Reports* 110, no. 6 (1995): 662–66.

Introduction

1. Jordan M. Rook et al., "Disparities in Screening for Substance Use Among Injured Adolescents," *JAMA Network Open* 7, no. 10 (2024): e2436371.

1. What Is This Thing Called Race?

1. A few recent books on this topic include Joseph L. Graves Jr. and Alan H. Goodman, *Racism, Not Race: Answers to Frequently Asked Questions* (Columbia University Press, 2021); David E. Bernstein, *Classified: The Untold Story of Racial Classification in America* (Bombardier, 2022); Richard W. Sussman, *The Myth of Race: The Troubling Persistence of an Unscientific Idea* (Harvard University Press, 2016); Alan H. Goodman, Yolanda T. Moses, and Joseph L. Jones, *Race: Are We So Different?*, 2nd ed. (Wiley-Blackwell, 2020); Angela Saini, *Superior: The Return of Race Science* (Beacon, 2019); Alondra Nelson, *The Social Life of DNA: Race, Reparations, and Reconciliation After the Genome* (Beacon, 2016); Dorothy Roberts, *Fatal

Invention: How Science, Politics, and Big Business Re-create Race in the Twenty-First Century (New Press, 2012).

2. Richard T. Schaefer, ed., *Encyclopedia of Race, Ethnicity, and Society* (Sage, 2008); Ellis Cashmore, ed., *Encyclopedia of Race and Ethnic Studies* (Routledge, 2004); John Stone, Rutledge M. Dennis, Polly S. Rizova, Anthony D. Smith, and Xiaoshuo Hou, eds., *The Wiley Blackwell Encyclopedia of Race, Ethnicity, and Nationalism* (Wiley, 2016); Patrick L. Mason, ed., *Encyclopedia of Race and Racism* (Macmillan, 2013).

3. Isabel Wilkerson, *Caste: The Origins of Our Discontents* (Random House, 2020).

4. Thierry Hoquet, "Biologization of Race and Racialization of the Human: Bernier, Buffon, Linnaeus," in *The Invention of Race*, ed. Nicolas Bancel, Thomas David, and Dominic Thomas (Routledge, 2014).

5. Nikole Hannah-Jones, *The 1619 Project: A New Origin Story* (One World, 2021).

6. Audrey Smedley, *Race in North America: Origin and Evolution of a Worldview* (Routledge, 2018).

7. Lyle N. McAlister, "Social Structure and Social Change in New Spain," *Hispanic American Historical Review* 43, no. 3 (1963): 349–70.

8. Christine B. Hickman, "The Devil and the One Drop Rule: Racial Categories, African Americans, and the US Census," *Michigan Law Review* 95 (1996): 1161–265.

9. Andrew J. Jolivette, ed., *Obama and the Biracial Factor: The Battle for a New American Majority* (Policy, 2012); Gregory John Leslie and David O. Sears, "The Heaviest Drop of Blood: Black Exceptionalism Among Multiracials," *Political Psychology* 43, no. 6 (2022): 1123–45.

10. Thomas Laqueur, "The Pocahontas Exception: America's Ancestor Obsession," *London Review of Books* 45, no. 7 (March 30, 2023), https://www.lrb.co.uk/the-paper/v45/n07/thomas-laqueur-the-pocahontas-exception.

11. Virginia R. Dominguez, *White by Definition: Social Classification in Creole Louisiana* (Rutgers University Press, 1993), 36–55.

12. Sharon M. Lee, "Racial Classifications in the US Census: 1890–1990," *Ethnic and Racial Studies* 16, no. 1 (1993): 75–94.

13. Daniel J. Friedman et al., "Race/Ethnicity and OMB Directive 15: Implications for State Public Health Practice," *American Journal of Public Health* 90, no. 11 (2000): 1714.

14. Clara E. Rodriguez, *Changing Race: Latinos, the Census, and the History of Ethnicity in the United States*, vol. 41 (New York University Press, 2000).

15. Office of Management and Budget, "Revisions to the Standards for the Classification of Federal Data on Race and Ethnicity," *Federal Register* 62, no. 210 (October 30, 1997), https://www.govinfo.gov/content/pkg/FR-1997-10-30/pdf/97-28653.pdf.

16. "Revisions to the Office of Management and Budget's Statistical Policy Directive No. 15: Standards for Maintaining, Collecting, and Presenting Federal Data on Race and Ethnicity. A Notice by the Management and Budget Office on 03/29/2024," *Federal Register*, https://www.federalregister.gov/d/2024-06469.

17. "U.S. Office of Management and Budget's Statistical Policy Directive No. 15: Standards for Maintaining, Collecting, and Presenting Federal Data on Race and Ethnicity," U.S. Office of Management and Budget, https://spd15revision.gov/.

18. Associated Press, "136 Variations of Brazilian Skin Colors," June 22, 2014, https://apnews.com/article/438c062613024c0c8f7908b485d12726.

19. Jo C. Phelan and Bruce G. Link, "Is Racism a Fundamental Cause of Inequalities in Health?," *Annual Review of Sociology* 41 (2015): 311–30.

20. William Darity and Samuel L. Myers, *Persistent Disparity* (Edward Elgar, 1998).

21. Troy Duster, "Race and Reification in Science," *Science* 307, no. 5712 (2005): 1050–51.

22. Maria Melchior et al., "À quand une prise en compte des disparités ethnoraciales vis-à-vis de l'infection à COVID-19 en France?," *Revue d'Épidémiologie et de Santé Publique* 69, no. 2 (2021): 96–98.

23. Défenseur des Droits, "Inégalités d'accès aux droits et discrimination en France," June 25 2020, https://www.defenseurdesdroits.fr/fr/etudes-et-recherches/2020/06/inegalites-dacces-aux-droits-et-discriminations-en-france.

24. Joan H. Fujimura et al., "Clines Without Classes: How to Make Sense of Human Variation," *Sociological Theory* 32, no. 3 (2014): 208–27.

25. Ann Gibbons, "Shedding Light on Skin Color," *Science* 346, no. 6212 (2014): 934–36.

26. Cosimo Posth et al., "Pleistocene Mitochondrial Genomes Suggest a Single Major Dispersal of Non-Africans and a Late Glacial Population Turnover in Europe," *Current Biology* 26, no. 6 (2016): 827–33.

27. Alon Keinan et al., "Measurement of the Human Allele Frequency Spectrum Demonstrates Greater Genetic Drift in East Asians Than in Europeans," *Nature Genetics* 39, no. 10 (2007): 1251–55.

28. Lorna G. Moore, "Human Genetic Adaptation to High Altitude," *High Altitude Medicine and Biology* 2, no. 2 (2001): 257–79.

29. Frédéric B. Piel et al., "Global Epidemiology of Sickle Haemoglobin in Neonates: A Contemporary Geostatistical Model-Based Map and Population Estimates," *Lancet* 381, no. 9861 (2013): 142–51.

30. Jocelyn Kaiser, "Geneticists Should Rethink How They Use Race and Ethnicity, Panel Urges," *Science*, March 14, 2023, https://www.science.org/content/article/geneticists-should-rethink-how-they-use-race-and-ethnicity-panel-urges.

31. Norman J. Sauer, "Forensic Anthropology and the Concept of Race: If Races Don't Exist, Why Are Forensic Anthropologists So Good at Identifying Them?," *Social Science and Medicine* 34, no. 2 (1992): 107–11.

32. Karen M. Tabb, "Changes in Racial Categorization Over Time and Health Status: An Examination of Multiracial Young Adults in the USA," *Ethnicity and Health* 21, no. 2 (2016): 146–57.

33. Atu Agawu et al., "Patterns of Change in Race Category in the Electronic Medical Record of a Pediatric Population," *JAMA Pediatrics* 177, no. 5 (2023): 536–39.

34. Carolyn A. Liebler et al., "America's Churning Races: Race and Ethnicity Response Changes Between Census 2000 and the 2010 Census," *Demography* 54, no. 1 (2017): 259–84.

35. Cyndy R. Snyder, Prince Z. Wang, and Anjali R. Truitt, "Multiracial Patient Experiences with Racial Microaggressions in Health Care Settings," *Journal of Patient-Centered Research and Reviews* 5, no. 3 (2018): 229.

36. Race, Ethnicity, and Genetics Working Group, "The Use of Racial, Ethnic, and Ancestral Categories in Human Genetics Research," *American Journal of Human Genetics* 77, no. 4 (2005): 519–32.

37. In fact, even the notion of a native Japanese population is complicated because there also exists an aboriginal Japanese population, the Ainu people.

38. Taylor Orth, "DNA Tests: Many Americans Report Surprises and New Connections," YouGov, February 24, 2022, https://today.yougov.com/topics /society/articles-reports/2022/02/24/dna-tests-many-americans-report -surprises-and-new-.

39. Anna C. F. Lewis et al., "Getting Genetic Ancestry Right for Science and Society," *Science* 376, no. 6590 (2022): 250–52.

40. Troy Duster, "Ancestry Testing and DNA: Uses, Limits—and Caveat Emptor," in *Genetics as Social Practice: Transdisciplinary Views on Science and Culture*, ed. Barbara Prainsack, Silke Schicktanz, and Gabriele Werner-Felmayer (Routledge, 2016).

41. Deborah A. Bolnick et al., "The Science and Business of Genetic Ancestry Testing," *Science* 318, no. 5849 (2007): 399–400.

42. Erin Aubry Kaplan, "Black Like I Thought I Was," *LA Weekly*, October 7, 2003.

43. C. F. Manski, J. Mullahy, and A. S. Venkataramani, "Using Measures of Race to Make Clinical Predictions: Decision Making, Patient Health, and Fairness," *Proceedings of the National Academy of Sciences of the United States of America* 120, no. 35 (2023): e2303370120.

44. Jay S. Kaufman, Joanna Merckx, and Richard S. Cooper, "Use of Racial and Ethnic Categories in Medical Testing and Diagnosis: Primum Non Nocere," *Clinical Chemistry* 67, no. 11 (2021): 1456–65.

45. Baz Dresisinger, "When Saying You're Black and Being Black Are Two Different Things," *Washington Post*, March 24, 2017, https://www.washingtonpost .com/opinions/when-saying-youre-black-and-being-black-are-two-different -things/2017/03/24/d41a6590-0a4b-11e7-93dc-00f9bdd74ed1_story.html.

46. Aaron Panofsky, Kushan Dasgupta, and Nicole Iturriaga, "How White Nationalists Mobilize Genetics: From Genetic Ancestry and Human Biodiversity to Counterscience and Metapolitics," *American Journal of Physical Anthropology* 175, no. 2 (2021): 387–98.

47. Jay S. Kaufman, "Ethical Dilemmas in Statistical Practice: The Problem of Race in Biomedicine," in *Mapping Race: A Critical Reader on Health Disparities Research*, ed. L. Gómez and N. López (Rutgers University Press, 2013).

2. Causality and the Fundamental Challenge of Observed Correlation

1. B. C. Kahan, S. Cro, F. Li, and M. O. Harhay, "Eliminating Ambiguous Treatment Effects Using Estimands," *American Journal of Epidemiology* 192, no. 6 (2023): 987–94.

2. Anders Huitfeldt, "Is Caviar a Risk Factor for Being a Millionaire?," *BMJ* 355 (2016): i6536.

3. Herbert L. Smith, "Some Thoughts on Causation as It Relates to Demography and Population Studies," *Population and Development Review* 29, no. 3 (2003): 459–69.

4. Catherine R. Lesko, Matthew P. Fox, and Jessie K. Edwards, "A Framework for Descriptive Epidemiology," *American Journal of Epidemiology* 191, no. 12 (2022): 2063–70.

5. Yan Li, Katherine E. Irimata, Yulei He, and Jennifer Parker, "Variable Inclusion Strategies Through Directed Acyclic Graphs to Adjust Health Surveys Subject to Selection Bias for Producing National Estimates," *Journal of Official Statistics* 38, no. 3 (2022): 875–900.

6. Graham Kalton, "Methods for Oversampling Rare Subpopulations in Social Surveys," *Survey Methodology* 35, no. 2 (2009): 125–41.

7. Julia Dressel and Hany Farid, "The Accuracy, Fairness, and Limits of Predicting Recidivism," *Science Advances* 4, no. 1 (2018): eaao5580.

8. Lars G. Hemkens et al., "Interpretation of Epidemiologic Studies Very Often Lacked Adequate Consideration of Confounding," *Journal of Clinical Epidemiology* 93 (2018): 94–102.

9. The formula for solving this problem analytically is actually rather complicated, so I obtained these numbers simply by having my computer flip millions of imaginary coins and counting the results.

10. Indeed, the word "confounding" in English is just a slightly archaic synonym for "confusion," and the words used in Romance languages for this same phenomenon are the cognates of "confusion": "confusion" in French, "confusión" in Spanish, and "confusão" in Portuguese, for example.

11. Technically, we expect the difference between the average age in the treated and the average age in the untreated to get closer to zero as the sample size of the trial gets larger. This is like the convergence to the expected 50 percent coin flip probability in the gambling game. This is why randomized trials require a sample size calculation before the trial begins to determine how many people are required to guarantee a predetermined degree of balance.

12. Bernie Devlin, Stephen E. Fienberg, Daniel P. Resnick, and Kathryn Roeder, eds., *Intelligence, Genes, and Success: Scientists Respond to the Bell Curve* (Springer Science and Business Media, 1997).

13. Tyler J. VanderWeele and Miguel A. Hernán, "Causal Effects and Natural Laws: Towards a Conceptualization of Causal Counterfactuals for Nonmanipulable Exposures, with Application to the Effects of Race and Sex," in *Causality: Statistical Perspectives and Applications*, ed. Walter A. Shewhart and Samuel S. Wilks (Wiley, 2012).

14. Select a random parent–child pair from the U.S. population and take the recorded race and sex from the parent's birth certificate and try to predict the race and sex recorded on the child's birth certificate. One will do a reasonably good job of predicting child race from a parent's race because most American children are racially concordant with their parents. Only about 1 percent of American children are adopted transracially, and more than 80 percent of U.S. marriages are racially concordant. In predicting the sex of a child from a parent's sex, however, one will only guess right about 50 percent of the time. Gretchen Livingston and Anna Brown, "Intermarriage in the U.S. 50 Years After Loving v. Virginia," Pew Research, May 18, 2017, https://www.pewresearch.org/social-trends/2017/05/18/intermarriage-in-the-u-s-50-years-after-loving-v-virginia/.

15. Robin Dembroff and Dee Payton, "Why We Shouldn't Compare Transracial to Transgender Identity," *Boston Review*, November 18, 2020, https://www.bostonreview.net/articles/robin-dembroff-dee-payton-breaking-analogy-between-race-and-gender/.

16. A German officer named Claus von Stauffenberg placed a bomb under the table during a meeting with Hitler at his military headquarters on July 20, 1944. Several attendees at the meeting were killed, but Hitler himself was partially shielded from the explosion by a solid-oak table leg and was therefore only slightly wounded. Alex Last, "The German Officer Who Tried to Kill Hitler," BBC, July 20, 2014, https://www.bbc.com/news/magazine-28330605.

17. He also shaved his head and spent up to half the day under an ultraviolet lamp. John Howard Griffin, *Black Like Me* (Houghton Mifflin, 1961).

18. Marti Loring and Brian Powell, "Gender, Race, and DSM-III: A Study of the Objectivity of Psychiatric Diagnostic Behavior," *Journal of Health and Social Behavior* 29 (1988): 1–22.

19. S. Michael Gaddis, ed., *Audit Studies: Behind the Scenes with Theory, Method, and Nuance* (Springer, 2018).

20. Marianne Bertrand and Sendhil Mullainathan, "Are Emily and Greg More Employable Than Lakisha and Jamal? A Field Experiment on Labor Market Discrimination," *American Economic Review* 94, no. 4 (2004): 991–1013.

21. Issa Kohler-Hausmann, "Eddie Murphy and the Dangers of Counterfactual Causal Thinking About Detecting Racial Discrimination," *Northwestern University Law Review* 113 (2018): 1163–227.

22. James J. Heckman, "Detecting Discrimination," *Journal of Economic Perspectives* 12, no. 2 (1998): 101–16.

23. The setup in this example is that the population has a mean of 100 and standard deviation of 10. Men have a mean of 100 and standard deviation of 11, whereas women have a mean of 100 and standard deviation of 9. To get the tail proportion in each group, find the Z-score, which is $Z = (X - \mu)/\sigma$. For men, $Z = 30/11 \approx 2.73$. For women, $Z = 30/9 \approx 3.33$. The area to the right of the Z-score for a normal distribution is the frequency of people exceeding that threshold. For men this is $1 - 0.9968 = 0.0032$, so 32 of every 10,000 men exceed this threshold. For women, $1 - 0.9994 = 0.0006$, which means that 6 of every 10,000 women exceed this threshold. This means that men will satisfy the criterion at a ratio of more than five to one, even when the groups have the same average ability.

24. Scott Jaschik, "What Larry Summers Said," *Inside Higher Education*, February 18, 2005, https://www.insidehighered.com/news/2005/02/18/what-larry-summers -said.

25. Knox H. Todd, Christi Deaton, Anne P. D'Adamo, and Leon Goe, "Ethnicity and Analgesic Practice," *Annals of Emergency Medicine* 35, no. 1 (2000): 11–16.

26. Robert S. White et al., "Multicenter Perioperative Outcomes Group Collaborators; Antiemetic Administration and Its Association with Race: A Retrospective Cohort Study," *Anesthesiology* 138 (2023): 587–601.

27. Neil Bhutta, Aurel Hizmo, and Daniel Ringo, "How Much Does Racial Bias Affect Mortgage Lending? Evidence from Human and Algorithmic Credit Decisions," FRB Philadelphia Consumer Finance Institute Working Paper, March 7, 2024, https://papers.ssrn.com/sol3/Papers.cfm?abstract_id=3887663.

28. Jay S. Kaufman, "Epidemiologic Analysis of Racial/Ethnic Disparities: Some Fundamental Issues and a Cautionary Example," *Social Science and Medicine* 66, no. 8 (2008): 1659–69.

29. Jay S. Kaufman and Richard S. Cooper, "Commentary: Considerations for Use of Racial/Ethnic Classification in Etiologic Research," *American Journal of Epidemiology* 154, no. 4 (2001): 291–98.

30. James S. Koopman, Carl P. Simon, and Chris P. Riolo, "When to Control Endemic Infections by Focusing on High-Risk Groups," *Epidemiology* 16 (2005): 621–27.

31. Miguel A. Hernán and Sarah L. Taubman, "Does Obesity Shorten Life? The Importance of Well-Defined Interventions to Answer Causal Questions," *International Journal of Obesity* 32, no. 3 (2008): S8–14.

32. Jay S. Kaufman and Richard S. Cooper, "Seeking Causal Explanations in Social Epidemiology," *American Journal of Epidemiology* 150, no. 2 (1999): 113–20.

33. Clark Glymour and Madelyn R. Glymour, "Commentary: Race and Sex Are Causes," *Epidemiology* 25, no. 4 (2014): 488–90.

34. Nancy Krieger, "On the Causal Interpretation of Race," *Epidemiology* 25, no. 6 (2014): 937.

3. Making Other Worlds

1. $(51 \times 3110792328) + (104 \times 9161031776) + (318 \times 26558529861) + (1200 \times 83113086000) + (8106 \times 78137518800)/(322273167) = 891.95$
2. $(50 \times 3110792328) + (93 \times 9161031776) + (246 \times 26558529861) + (1059 \times 83113086000) + (7485 \times 78137518800)/(322273167) = 800.31$
3. Federal government statistics such as those from the Centers for Disease Control and Prevention use five-year age categories, whereas I used much wider categories, allowing for some remaining imbalance within the groups in my calculation.
4. Thomas J. Bollyky et al., "Assessing COVID-19 Pandemic Policies and Behaviours and Their Economic and Educational Trade-Offs Across US States from Jan 1, 2020, to July 31, 2022: An Observational Analysis," *Lancet* 401, no. 10385 (2023): 1341–60.
5. R. N. Anderson and H. M. Rosenberg, "Age Standardization of Death Rates: Implementation of the Year 2000 Standard," *National Vital Statistics Reports* 47, no. 3 (1998): 1–20.
6. Paul D. Sorlie et al., "Age-Adjusted Death Rates: Consequences of the Year 2000 Standard," *Annals of Epidemiology* 9, no. 2 (1999): 93–100.
7. KFF, "Total Deaths by Race/Ethnicity," 2022, https://www.kff.org/other/state -indicator/death-rate-by-raceethnicity/.
8. Hoben Thomas and Thomas P. Hettmansperger, "Risk Ratios and Scanlan's HRX," *Journal of Statistical Distributions and Applications* 4, no. 1 (2017): 1–15.
9. Centers for Disease Control and Prevention, National Center for Health Statistics, "National Vital Statistics System, Mortality 1999–2020 on CDC WONDER Online Database, Released in 2021," accessed December 1, 2022, http://wonder .cdc.gov/ucd-icd10.html. Data are from the Multiple Cause of Death Files, 1999–2020, as compiled from data provided by the fifty-seven vital statistics jurisdictions through the Vital Statistics Cooperative Program.
10. Nancy Krieger and David R. Williams, "Changing to the 2000 Standard Million: Are Declining Racial/Ethnic and Socioeconomic Inequalities in Health Real Progress or Statistical Illusion?," *American Journal of Public Health* 91, no. 8 (2001): 1209–13.
11. Chik Collins, "Austerity and Mortality in Spain: The Perils of Overcorrecting an Analytic Mistake," *American Journal of Public Health* 109, no. 7 (2019): 963–65.
12. David Leonhardt, "Covid and Race," *New York Times*, June 9, 2022, https://www .nytimes.com/2022/06/09/briefing/covid-race-deaths-america.html.
13. Katelyn Jetelina, "The Morning Today Is . . . Wrong," Your Local Epidemiologist, June 9, 2022, https://yourlocalepidemiologist.substack.com/p/the-morning -today-iswrong.
14. Gregg Gonsalves (@greggonsalves), "This is irresponsible, wrong and is misinformation—full stop. There is no excuse. Why does it happen? Because no

one fact-checks this man, no one checks his analysis. It's inexcusable and does tremendous damage to real people and to the pandemic response," Twitter, June 9, 2022; Ann Batenburg (@AnnBatenburg), "It's time to take @DLeonhardt off the COVID beat. He's done enough harm. It has been obvious that he is not an expert in the field, and we see clearly the limits of journalism without expertise. So, get someone who what they are talking about," Twitter, June 9, 2022.

15. David Leonhardt (@DLeonhardt), "I agree that age is part of the story. I disagree that it overwhelms everything else. The story here is real: Covid killed a much larger percentage of Black of Latino Americans than white Americans during the pandemic's first year. During the past year, Covid has killed a higher percentage of white Americans than Black, Latino or Asian Americans," Twitter, June 9, 2022.

16. Gregg Gonsalves (@gregggonsalves), "David stop. You succumbed to Simpson's paradox and were wrong. Have the common decency to say it. Your analysis was flawed. People have pointed it out and it's a first-year public health student mistake. Now you're doubling down, and doing the 'left' is after me shtick. It's so deeply disingenuous of you, and yes, manipulative," Twitter, June 9, 2022.

17. Nazrul Islam and Dmitri A. Jdanov, "Age and Sex Adjustments Are Critical When Comparing Death Rates," *BMJ* 381 (2023): 845.

18. Katherine A. Thurber et al., "Reflection on Modern Methods: Statistical, Policy and Ethical Implications of Using Age-Standardized Health Indicators to Quantify Inequities," *International Journal of Epidemiology* 51, no. 1 (2022): 324–33.

19. E. Arias, B. Tejada-Vera, K. D. Kochanek, and F. B. Ahmad, "Provisional Life Expectancy Estimates for 2021," Vital Statistics Rapid Release, no. 23, National Center for Health Statistics, August 2022, https://www.cdc.gov/nchs/data/vsrr/vsrr023.pdf.

20. Sam Harper, Richard F. MacLehose, and Jay S. Kaufman, "Trends in the Black-White Life Expectancy Gap Among US States, 1990–2009," *Health Affairs* 33, no. 8 (2014): 1375–82.

21. Héctor Pifarré i Arolas et al., "US Racial–Ethnic Mortality Gap Adjusted for Population Structure," *Epidemiology* 34, no. 3 (2023): 402–10.

22. Faced with any argument in the form "if A, then B," rejection of A means that we can infer nothing whatsoever about B, and so posing an impossible A makes consideration of B all but moot. This logic is expressed poignantly by the character Cassandra in the 1992 film *Wayne's World* with the expression: "If a frog had wings, it wouldn't bump its ass when it hopped." Urban Dictionary, "if a frog had wings," March 26, 2007, https://www.urbandictionary.com/define.php?term=if a frog had wings.

23. CensusScope, "Percent Black/African American Ranking, 2000," https://censusscope.org/us/rank_race_blackafricanamerican.html.

24. Statista, "Death Rates from COVID-19 in the United States as of March 10, 2023, by State," March 28, 2023, https://www.statista.com/statistics/1109011/coronavirus-covid19-death-rates-us-by-state/.

25. RPubs, "David Leonhardt Is Correct About the 'Flip' in COVID-19 Racial Disparities," https://rpubs.com/random_critical_analysis/covid_racial_disparities _flipped; Akilah Johnson and Dan Keathing, "Whites Now More Likely to Die from Covid Than Blacks: Why the Pandemic Shifted," *Washington Post*, October 19, 2022, https://www.washingtonpost.com/health/2022/10/19/covid-deaths-us-race/.
26. David Leonhardt, "A Public Health Success Story," *New York Times*, October 4, 2022, https://www.nytimes.com/2022/10/04/briefing/covid-race-gaps.html.
27. Dielle J. Lundberg et al., "COVID-19 Mortality by Race and Ethnicity in US Metropolitan and Nonmetropolitan Areas, March 2020 to February 2022," *JAMA Network Open* 6, no. 5 (2023): e2311098.

4. Crude Versus Adjusted Racial and Ethnic Comparisons

1. In the Romance languages, like French and Spanish, the word "confusion" is still used for this same statistical phenomenon. The more archaic English word "confounding" did not become commonly used for this purpose until the latter half of the twentieth century. See Alfredo Morabia, "History of the Modern Epidemiological Concept of Confounding," *Journal of Epidemiology and Community Health* 65, no. 4 (2011): 297–300.
2. Just think about a randomized trial of antimalarial drugs in which participants are given mefloquine or placebo based on a coin flip. Because of the randomization, all traits of the participants will be equally distributed in the treatment and placebo groups, and thus one can expect no confounding. However, if we conduct this same study among Yorubas in Nigeria and among Inuit in northern Canada, there is no reason to expect that the treatment effects will be the same across these two groups. Indeed, we are certain to see no effect in the Inuit because malarial mosquitos do not exist in that environment. Therefore, the absence of confounding does not imply that treatment effects will be the same across racial or ethnic groups. Rather, these groups can reside in different environments, and these differing environments can cause the treatment to have distinct effects, a variation that epidemiologists call "effect measure modification" and economists call "effect heterogeneity."
3. This might seem to contradict the skepticism expressed over age adjustment in the *New York Times* example in chapter 3, but in that case, the different age distribution was a consequence of the same differential treatment by race that the study was intending to document. In the case of Mexican American versus Cuban American age structure differences, it has much less to do with racism in the United States and more to do with political history and social history within each country and the history of immigration from each country to the United States, including the different factors that drive immigration from each

sending country. Mexico also has a higher fertility rate than Cuba and a lower life expectancy, leading to an older age structure in Cuba as the sending country before even considering selection into immigration.

4. Nirmal K. Sampathkumar et al., "Widespread Sex Dimorphism in Aging and Age-Related Diseases," *Human Genetics* 139, no. 3 (2020): 333–56.

5. Paula Braveman and Sofia Gruskin, "Defining Equity in Health," *Journal of Epidemiology and Community Health* 57, no. 4 (2003): 254–58.

6. Jay S. Kaufman, "Chapter 4. Ethical Dilemmas in Statistical Practice: The Problem of Race in Biomedicine," in *Mapping "Race": Critical Approaches to Health Disparities Research*, ed. Laura E. Gómez and Nancy López (Rutgers University Press, 2013).

7. Amartya Sen, "What Do We Want from a Theory of Justice?," *Journal of Philosophy* 103, no. 5 (2006): 215–38.

8. Gary S. Becker, *The Economics of Discrimination* (University of Chicago Press, 2010); Luca Oneto and Silvia Chiappa, "Fairness in Machine Learning," in *Recent Trends in Learning from Data* (Springer, 2020).

9. Brian D. Smedley, Adrienne Y. Stith, and Alan R. Nelson, eds., *Unequal Treatment: Confronting Racial and Ethnic Disparities in Health Care* (National Academies Press, 2003).

10. Naihua Duan et al., "Disparities in Defining Disparities: Statistical Conceptual Frameworks," *Statistics in Medicine* 27, no. 20 (2008): 3941–56.

11. Christopher S. Lathan, Bridget A. Neville, and Craig C. Earle, "The Effect of Race on Invasive Staging and Surgery in Non–Small-Cell Lung Cancer," *Journal of Clinical Oncology* 24, no. 3 (2006): 413–18.

12. Samuel Cykert et al., "Factors Associated with Decisions to Undergo Surgery Among Patients with Newly Diagnosed Early-Stage Lung Cancer," *JAMA* 303, no. 23 (2010): 2368–76.

13. Sandra Susan Smith, "Race and Trust," *Annual Review of Sociology* 36 (2010): 453–75.

14. Katherine A. Thurber et al., "Reflection on Modern Methods: Statistical, Policy and Ethical Implications of Using Age-Standardized Health Indicators to Quantify Inequities," *International Journal of Epidemiology* 51, no. 1 (2022): 324–33.

15. Matthew Chingos, "Breaking the Curve: Promises and Pitfalls of Using NAEP Data to Assess the State Role in Student Achievement," Urban Institute, 2016, https://www.urban.org/research/publication/breaking-curve-promises-and-pitfalls-using-naep-data-assess-state-role-student-achievement.

16. Urban.org., "America's Gradebook: How Does Your State Stack Up?," https://apps.urban.org/features/naep/.

17. Wiktionary, "Soft Bigotry of Low Expectations," https://en.wiktionary.org/wiki/soft_bigotry_of_low_expectations.

18. Mercedes De Onis and Francesco Branca, "Childhood Stunting: A Global Perspective," *Maternal and Child Nutrition* 12 (2016): 12–26.

19. World Health Organization Multicentre Growth Reference Study Group and Mercedes de Onis, "Enrolment and Baseline Characteristics in the WHO Multicentre Growth Reference Study," *Acta Paediatrica* 95 (2006): 7–15.

20. S. V. Subramanian, Omar Karlsson, and Rockli Kim, "Revisiting the Stunting Metric for Monitoring and Evaluating Nutrition Policies," *Lancet Global Health* 10, no. 2 (2022): e179–80.

21. Omar Karlsson, Rockli Kim, Barry Bogin, and S. V. Subramanian, "Maternal Height-Standardized Prevalence of Stunting in 67 Low- and Middle-Income Countries," *Journal of Epidemiology* 32, no. 7 (2022): 337–44.

22. John Gramlich, "What the Data Says About Crime in the U.S.," Pew Research Center, April 24, 2024, https://www.pewresearch.org/short-reads/2024/04/24/what-the-data-says-about-crime-in-the-us/.

23. Maxim Massenkoff and Aaron Chalfin, "Activity-Adjusted Crime Rates Show That Public Safety Worsened in 2020," *Proceedings of the National Academy of Sciences* 119, no. 46 (2022): e2208598119.

24. Emily Leslie and Riley Wilson, "Sheltering in Place and Domestic Violence: Evidence from Calls for Service During COVID-19," *Journal of Public Economics* 189 (2020): 104241.

25. Jean A. McDougall et al., "Racial and Ethnic Disparities in Cervical Cancer Incidence Rates in the United States, 1992–2003," *Cancer Causes and Control* 18, no. 10 (2007): 1175–86; Divya A. Patel et al., "A Population-Based Study of Racial and Ethnic Differences in Survival Among Women with Invasive Cervical Cancer: Analysis of Surveillance, Epidemiology, and End Results Data," *Gynecologic Oncology* 97, no. 2 (2005): 550–58.

26. Anna L. Beavis, Patti E. Gravitt, and Anne F. Rositch, "Hysterectomy-Corrected Cervical Cancer Mortality Rates Reveal a Larger Racial Disparity in the United States," *Cancer* 123, no. 6 (2017): 1044–50.

27. How did the authors calculate that the previously uncorrected surveillance had underestimated the racial mortality disparity by over 40 percent? The calculation is a bit convoluted, but this is where their estimate comes from. The uncorrected disparity was 5.7 per 100,000 Black women per year divided by 3.2 per 100,000 white women per year, or a ratio of 1.78. Thus, the Black excess had been 78 percent. The corrected disparity became 10.1 per 100,000 Black women per year divided by 4.7 per 100,000 white women per year, a ratio of 2.15, which is a 115 percent Black excess. The authors calculated that 115 percent/78 percent = 1.47, so that the updated disparity was 47 percent larger. You could come to the same conclusion by comparing the absolute disparities instead of the ratios. The previous racial disparity was 5.7 − 3.2 = 2.5 excess cases per 100,000 Black women per year, and the updated disparity is 10.1 − 4.7 = 5.4 excess cases per 100,000 Black women per year; 2.5 is 46 percent as large as 5.4, so the conclusion is roughly the same.

28. Jiayao Lei et al., "HPV Vaccination and the Risk of Invasive Cervical Cancer," *New England Journal of Medicine* 383, no. 14 (2020): 1340–48.

29. Jacqueline Howard, "Cervical Cancer Death Rates Are Much Higher Than Thought, Study Says," CNN, January 25, 2017, https://edition.cnn.com/2017/01/23/health/cervical-cancer-death-study/index.html.

30. Clyde Hughes, "Cervical Cancer Death Rates Shockingly Underestimated," Newsmax, January 24, 2017, https://www.newsmax.com/thewire/cervical-cancer-death-rates-underestimated/2017/01/24/id/770113/.

31. Miguel A. Hernán, Wei Wang, and David E. Leaf, "Target Trial Emulation: A Framework for Causal Inference from Observational Data," *JAMA* 328, no. 24 (2022): 2446–47.

5. Conditional Disparities Are the Devil's Playground

1. Jonas H. Ellenberg, "Selection Bias in Observational and Experimental Studies," *Statistics in Medicine* 13, no. 5–7 (1994): 557–67.

2. Christopher Winship and Robert D. Mare, "Models for Sample Selection Bias," *Annual Review of Sociology* 18 (1992): 327–50.

3. Judea Pearl, "Causal Diagrams for Empirical Research," *Biometrika* 82, no. 4 (1995): 669–88.

4. Miguel A. Hernán, Sonia Hernández-Díaz, and James M. Robins, "A Structural Approach to Selection Bias," *Epidemiology* 15 (2004): 615–25.

5. Miguel A. Hernán, "Invited Commentary: Selection Bias Without Colliders," *American Journal of Epidemiology* 185, no. 11 (2017): 1048–50.

6. M. Maria Glymour, "Using Causal Diagrams to Understand Common Problems in Social Epidemiology," in *Methods in Social Epidemiology*, ed. J. M. Oakes and J. S. Kaufman (Wiley, 2006).

7. Gareth J. Griffith et al., "Collider Bias Undermines Our Understanding of COVID-19 Disease Risk and Severity," *Nature Communications* 11, no. 1 (2020): 1–12.

8. Greg R. Alexander et al., "Racial Differences in the Relation of Birth Weight and Gestational Age to Neonatal Mortality," *Public Health Reports* 100, no. 5 (1985): 539–47.

9. J. Yerushalmy, "The Relationship of Parents' Cigarette Smoking to Outcome of Pregnancy—Implications as to the Problem of Inferring Causation from Observed Associations," *American Journal of Epidemiology* 93, no. 6 (1971): 443–56.

10. Allen Wilcox and Ian Russell, "Why Small Black Infants Have a Lower Mortality Rate Than Small White Infants: The Case for Population-Specific Standards for Birth Weight," *Journal of Pediatrics* 116, no. 1 (1990): 7–10.

11. Allen J. Wilcox, "On the Importance—and the Unimportance—of Birthweight," *International Journal of Epidemiology* 30, no. 6 (2001): 1233–41.

12. Ana Migone et al., "Gestational Duration and Birthweight in White, Black and Mixed-Race Babies," *Paediatric and Perinatal Epidemiology* 5, no. 4 (1991): 378–91.

13. Sonia Hernández-Díaz, Enrique F. Schisterman, and Miguel A. Hernán, "The Birth Weight 'Paradox' Uncovered?," *American Journal of Epidemiology* 164, no. 11 (2006): 1115–20.

14. Stephen R. Cole et al., "Illustrating Bias due to Conditioning on a Collider," *International Journal of Epidemiology* 39, no. 2 (2010): 417–20.

15. Mark A. Klebanoff, "Crossing Birth–Weight–Specific Mortality Curves: How a Puzzling Clinical Observation Led to an Important Advance in Epidemiologic Methods," *American Journal of Epidemiology* 192, no. 11 (2023): 1793–96.

16. Bohao Wu et al., "Birth-Based vs Fetuses-at-Risk Approaches for Assessing Neonatal Mortality Rate by Race," *JAMA Pediatrics* 177, no. 6 (2023): 633–35.

17. Hailey R. Banack and Jay S. Kaufman, "The Obesity Paradox: Understanding the Effect of Obesity on Mortality Among Individuals with Cardiovascular Disease," *Preventive Medicine* 62 (2014): 96–102.

18. Sam Levin, "'It Never Stops': Killings by US Police Reach Record High in 2022," *The Guardian*, January 6, 2023, https://www.theguardian.com/us-news/2023/jan/06/us-police-killings-record-number-2022.

19. Dean Knox and Jonathan Mummolo, "Making Inferences About Racial Disparities in Police Violence," *Proceedings of the National Academy of Sciences* 117, no. 3 (2020): 1261–62.

20. Roland G. Fryer Jr., "An Empirical Analysis of Racial Differences in Police Use of Force," *Journal of Political Economy* 127, no. 3 (2019): 1210–61.

21. Fryer, "An Empirical Analysis of Racial Differences in Police Use of Force," 1212.

22. Robert Silk, "Ski Industry Examines Its Lack of Diversity," *Travel Weekly*, July 24, 2020, https://www.travelweekly.com/Travel-News/Travel-Agent-Issues/Ski-industry-examines-lack-of-diversity.

23. Fryer, "An Empirical Analysis of Racial Differences in Police Use of Force," 1214.

24. "How a Controversial Study Found That Police Are More Likely to Shoot Whites, Not Blacks," *Washington Post*, July 13, 2016, https://www.washingtonpost.com/news/wonk/wp/2016/07/13/why-a-massive-new-study-on-police-shootings-of-whites-and-blacks-is-so-controversial/.

25. Valerie Richardson, "No Racial Bias in Police Shootings, Study by Harvard Professor Shows," *Washington Times*, July 11, 2016, https://www.washingtontimes.com/news/2016/jul/11/no-racial-bias-police-shootings-study-harvard-prof/.

26. Quoctrung Bui and Amanda Cox, "Surprising New Evidence Shows Bias in Police Use of Force but Not in Shootings," *New York Times*, July 12, 2016, https://www.nytimes.com/2016/07/12/upshot/surprising-new-evidence-shows-bias-in-police-use-of-force-but-not-in-shootings.html.

27. Dean Knox, Will Lowe, and Jonathan Mummolo, "Administrative Records Mask Racially Biased Policing," *American Political Science Review* 114, no. 3 (2020): 619–37.

28. Steven N. Durlauf and James J. Heckman, "An Empirical Analysis of Racial Differences in Police Use of Force: A Comment," *Journal of Political Economy* 128, no. 10 (2020): 3998–4002.

29. Roland G. Fryer Jr., "An Empirical Analysis of Racial Differences in Police Use of Force: A Response," *Journal of Political Economy* 128, no. 10 (2020): 4003–8.

30. Here is one recent interview example in which Fryer describes his paper as documenting an absence of racial bias in police shootings, in contradiction to his response to Durlauf and Heckman: Coleman Hughes, "Overcoming the Odds with Roland Fryer," June 5, 2022, https://www.youtube.com/watch?v=qNClcjDOVmk.

31. Robert VerBruggen, "Fatal Police Shootings and Race: A Review of the Evidence and Suggestions for Future Research," *Manhattan Institute Report* (2022): 1–32.

32. David J. Johnson et al., "Officer Characteristics and Racial Disparities in Fatal Officer-Involved Shootings," *Proceedings of the National Academy of Sciences* 116, no. 32 (2019): 15877–82.

33. Dean Knox and Jonathan Mummolo, "Making Inferences About Racial Disparities in Police Violence," *Proceedings of the National Academy of Sciences* 117, no. 3 (2020): 1261–62.

34. Dean Knox and Jonathan Mummolo, "It Took Us Months to Contest a Flawed Study on Police Bias. Here's Why That's Dangerous," *Washington Post*, January 28, 2020, https://www.washingtonpost.com/opinions/2020/01/28/it-took-us -months-contest-flawed-study-police-bias-heres-why-thats-dangerous/.

35. "Retraction for Johnson et al., Officer Characteristics and Racial Disparities in Fatal Officer-Involved Shootings," *Proceedings of the National Academy of Sciences of the United States of America* 117 (2020): 18130, https://doi.org/10.1073 /pnas.2014148117.

36. Anna Fry et al., "Comparison of Sociodemographic and Health-Related Characteristics of UK Biobank Participants with Those of the General Population," *American Journal of Epidemiology* 186, no. 9 (2017): 1026–34.

37. "UK Biobank . . . Only Just Getting into Its Stride," UK Biobank, November 4, 2022, https://www.ukbiobank.ac.uk/explore-your-participation/stay-involved /2022-newsletter/uk-biobank-only-just-getting-into-its-stride.

38. Jukka Savolainen, "How Social Science Research Is Censored to Push a Progressive Agenda," *National Post*, June 27, 2023, https://nationalpost.com/opinion /how-social-science-research-is-policed-to-push-a-progressive-agenda.

39. Douglas S. Massey and Mary C. Waters, "Scientific Versus Public Debates: A PNAS Case Study," *Proceedings of the National Academy of Sciences* 117, no. 31 (2020): 18135–36.

40. Heather Mac Donald, "The Myth of Systemic Police Racism," *Wall Street Journal*, June 2, 2020.
41. Marian Jarlenski et al., "Association of Race with Urine Toxicology Testing Among Pregnant Patients During Labor and Delivery," *JAMA Health Forum* 4 (2023): e230441, https://www.doi.org/10.1001/jamahealthforum.2023.0441.
42. Jacqueline E. Rudolph, Catherine R. Lesko, and Ashley I. Naimi, "Causal Inference in the Face of Competing Events," *Current Epidemiology Reports* 7, no. 3 (2020): 125–31.
43. G. Fairclough, "Smoking Can Help Czech Economy, Philip Morris–Little Report Says," *Wall Street Journal*, July 17, 2001, http://online.wsj.com/article/SB995230746855683470.html.
44. Jennifer Weuve et al., "Accounting for Bias due to Selective Attrition: The Example of Smoking and Cognitive Decline," *Epidemiology* 23, no. 1 (2012): 119–28.
45. Elizabeth Arias and Mortality Statistics Branch, "Race Crossover in Longevity," in *Encyclopedia of Gerontology and Population Aging* (Springer, 2019).
46. Steven D. Stovitz, Hailey R. Banack, and Jay S. Kaufman, "'Depletion of the Susceptibles' Taught Through a Story, a Table and Basic Arithmetic," *BMJ Evidence-Based Medicine* 23, no. 5 (2018): 199.
47. W. Dana Flanders and Mitchel Klein, "Properties of 2 Counterfactual Effect Definitions of a Point Exposure," *Epidemiology* 18 (2007): 453–60.
48. Jonathan Yinhao Huang, "Representativeness Is Not Representative: Addressing Major Inferential Threats in the UK Biobank and Other Big Data Repositories," *Epidemiology* 32, no. 2 (2021): 189–93.

6. The Mismeasure of Man

1. Stephen Jay Gould, *The Mismeasure of Man* (Norton, 1981).
2. James R. Flynn, *What Is Intelligence? Beyond the Flynn Effect* (Cambridge University Press, 2007).
3. Sharon I. Kirkpatrick et al., "Best Practices for Conducting and Interpreting Studies to Validate Self-Report Dietary Assessment Methods," *Journal of the Academy of Nutrition and Dietetics* 119, no. 11 (2019): 1801–16.
4. James M. Hodge et al., "Validation of Self-Reported Height and Weight in a Large, Nationwide Cohort of US Adults," *PloS One* 15, no. 4 (2020): e0231229.
5. "Pap smear" is actually slang for the test devised by the Greek doctor Georgios Papanikolaou in the years prior to World War II. The definitive publication was: George N. Papanicolaou and Herbert F. Traut, "The Diagnostic Value of Vaginal Smears in Carcinoma of the Uterus," *American Journal of Obstetrics and Gynecology* 42, no. 2 (1941): 193–206.

6. Marie-Hélène Mayrand et al., "Human Papillomavirus DNA Versus Papanicolaou Screening Tests for Cervical Cancer," *New England Journal of Medicine* 357, no. 16 (2007): 1579–88.

7. Jay S. Kaufman, "How Inconsistencies in Racial Classification Demystify the Race Construct in Public Health Statistics," *Epidemiology* 10 (1999): 101–3.

8. Steven Hitlin, J. Scott Brown, and Glen H. Elder Jr., "Racial Self-Categorization in Adolescence: Multiracial Development and Social Pathways," *Child Development* 77, no. 5 (2006): 1298–308; Luisa Farah Schwartzman, "Does Money Whiten? Intergenerational Changes in Racial Classification in Brazil," *American Sociological Review* 72, no. 6 (2007): 940–63.

9. Pew Research Center, "What Census Calls Us," February 6, 2020, http://www.pewsocialtrends.org/interactives/multiracial-timeline/.

10. Salvador Contreras, "For Economic Advantage or Something Else? A Case for Racial Identification Switching," *Review of Black Political Economy* 43, no. 3–4 (2016): 301–23.

11. David E. Bernstein, *Classified: The Untold Story of Racial Classification in America* (Bombardier, 2022), 87.

12. Neda Maghbouleh, Ariela Schachter, and René D. Flores, "Middle Eastern and North African Americans May Not Be Perceived, Nor Perceive Themselves, to Be White," *Proceedings of the National Academy of Sciences* 119, no. 7 (2022): e2117940119.

13. Lynn B. Jorde and Michael J. Bamshad, "Genetic Ancestry Testing: What Is It and Why Is It Important?," *JAMA* 323, no. 11 (2020): 1089–90.

14. Noah A. Rosenberg et al., "Genetic Structure of Human Populations," *Science* 298, no. 5602 (2002): 2381–85.

15. Mari Nelis et al., "Genetic Structure of Europeans: A View from the North–East," *PloS One* 4, no. 5 (2009): e5472.

16. Stephen Leslie et al., "The Fine-Scale Genetic Structure of the British Population," *Nature* 519, no. 7543 (2015): 309–14.

17. Ruby Jo Reeves Kennedy, "Single or Triple Melting-Pot? Intermarriage in New Haven, 1870–1950," *American Journal of Sociology* 58, no. 1 (1952): 56–59.

18. Pew Research, "Interfaith Marriage Is Common in U.S., Particularly Among the Recently Wed," June 2, 2015, https://www.pewresearch.org/short-reads/2015/06/02/interfaith-marriage/.

19. Anna C. F. Lewis et al., "Getting Genetic Ancestry Right for Science and Society," *Science* 376, no. 6590 (2022): 250–52.

20. Yi Huang et al., "Global, Regional, and National Burden of Neurological Disorders in 204 Countries and Territories Worldwide," *Journal of Global Health* 13 (2023), https://jogh.org/2023/jogh-13-04160.

21. Erin Aubry Kaplan, "Black Like I Thought I Was," *LA Weekly*, 2003, https://www.laweekly.com/black-like-i-thought-i-was/.

22. Anne M. Huml et al., "Consistency of Direct-to-Consumer Genetic Testing Results Among Identical Twins," *American Journal of Medicine* 133, no. 1 (2020): 143–46.
23. Ruth H. Keogh et al., "STRATOS Guidance Document on Measurement Error and Misclassification of Variables in Observational Epidemiology: Part 1—Basic Theory and Simple Methods of Adjustment," *Statistics in Medicine* 39, no. 16 (2020): 2197–231.
24. Physics World, "In Praise of Lord Kelvin," December 17, 2007, https://physicsworld.com/a/in-praise-of-lord-kelvin/.
25. Nancy López et al., "What's Your 'Street Race'? Leveraging Multidimensional Measures of Race and Intersectionality for Examining Physical and Mental Health Status Among Latinxs," *Sociology of Race and Ethnicity* 4, no. 1 (2018): 49–66.
26. Victoria E. Sosina and Aliya Saperstein, "Reflecting Race and Status: The Dynamics of Material Hardship and How People Are Perceived," *Socius* 8 (2022): 23780231221124578.
27. Andrew M. Penner and Aliya Saperstein, "Disentangling the Effects of Racial Self-Identification and Classification by Others: The Case of Arrest," *Demography* 52, no. 3 (2015): 1017–24.
28. Emma Pierson et al., "A Large-Scale Analysis of Racial Disparities in Police Stops Across the United States," *Nature Human Behaviour* 4, no. 7 (2020): 736–45.
29. Aaron Panofsky, Kushan Dasgupta, and Nicole Iturriaga, "How White Nationalists Mobilize Genetics: From Genetic Ancestry and Human Biodiversity to Counterscience and Metapolitics," *American Journal of Physical Anthropology* 175, no. 2 (2021): 387–98.
30. Sasha Shen Johfre, Aliya Saperstein, and Jill A. Hollenbach, "Measuring Race and Ancestry in the Age of Genetic Testing," *Demography* 58, no. 3 (2021): 785–810.
31. Bernstein, *Classified*, 114.
32. Jonathan Kahn, "The Legal Weaponization of Racialized DNA: A New Genetic Politics of Affirmative Action," *Georgetown Journal of Law and Modern Critical Race Perspectives* 13 (2021): 187.
33. Mathew R. Birnbaum et al., "Evaluation of Hair Density in Different Ethnicities in a Healthy American Population Using Quantitative Trichoscopic Analysis," *Skin Appendage Disorders* 4, no. 4 (2018): 304–7.
34. Erika E. Lynn-Green et al., "Variations in How Medical Researchers Report Patient Demographics: A Retrospective Analysis of Published Articles," *Eclinicalmedicine* 58, April 28, 2023, https://www.thelancet.com/journals/eclinm/article/PIIS2589-5370(23)00080-9/fulltext.
35. Andrew S. Levey and Lesley A. Inker, "Assessment of Glomerular Filtration Rate in Health and Disease: A State of the Art Review," *Clinical Pharmacology and Therapeutics* 102, no. 3 (2017): 405–19.

36. Andrew S. Levey et al., "A More Accurate Method to Estimate Glomerular Filtration Rate from Serum Creatinine: A New Prediction Equation," *Annals of Internal Medicine* 130, no. 6 (1999): 461–70.

37. The original correction factor was 18 percent, but the formula was simplified in 2006 and the correction factor adjusted to 21 percent. Lesley A. Stevens et al., "Assessing Kidney Function—Measured and Estimated Glomerular Filtration Rate," *New England Journal of Medicine* 354, no. 23 (2006): 2473–83.

38. Heather Morris and Sumit Mohan, "Using Race in the Estimation of Glomerular Filtration Rates: Time for a Reversal?," *Current Opinion in Nephrology and Hypertension* 29, no. 2 (2020): 227–31.

39. Haute Autorité de Santé, https://www.has-sante.fr/jcms/c_1064297/fr/evaluation-du-debit-de-filtration-glomerulaire-et-du-dosage-de-la-creatininemie-dans-le-diagnostic-de-la-maladie-renale-chronique-chez-l-adulte-rapport-d-evaluation.

40. "Clearance de la Créatinine: Formule CKD-EPI," http://medicalcul.free.fr/ckdepi.html.

41. Priya Vart et al., "Effectiveness and Safety of Dapagliflozin for Black and White Patients with Chronic Kidney Disease in North and South America: A Secondary Analysis of a Randomized Clinical Trial," *JAMA Network Open* 6, no. 4 (2023): e2310877, https://www.doi.org/10.1001/jamanetworkopen.2023.10877.

7. Proxies and Predictions

1. Statista, "Resident Population in New York from 1960 to 2023," October 28, 2024, https://www.statista.com/statistics/206267/resident-population-in-new-york/.

2. Lisa Bowleg and Greta Bauer, "Invited Reflection: Quantifying Intersectionality," *Psychology of Women Quarterly* 40, no. 3 (2016): 337–41.

3. Sander Greenland, "Summarization, Smoothing, and Inference in Epidemiologic Analysis," *Scandinavian Journal of Social Medicine* 21, no. 4 (1993): 227–32.

4. Amy Earley et al., "Estimating Equations for Glomerular Filtration Rate in the Era of Creatinine Standardization: A Systematic Review," *Annals of Internal Medicine* 156, no. 11 (2012): 785–95.

5. Andrew S. Levey et al., "A More Accurate Method to Estimate Glomerular Filtration Rate from Serum Creatinine: A New Prediction Equation," *Annals of Internal Medicine* 130, no. 6 (1999): 461–70.

6. Andrew S. Levey et al., "A New Equation to Estimate Glomerular Filtration Rate," *Annals of Internal Medicine* 150, no. 9 (2009): 604–12.

7. Levey et al., "A More Accurate Method to Estimate Glomerular Filtration Rate from Serum Creatinine," 464.

8. S. H. Cohn et al., "Body Elemental Composition: Comparison Between Black and White Adults," *American Journal of Physiology-Endocrinology and Metabolism* 232, no. 4 (1977): E419.

9. David W. Harsha, Ralph R. Frerichs, and Gerald S. Berenson, "Densitometry and Anthropometry of Black and White Children," *Human Biology* 50 (1978): 261–80.

10. J. G. Worrall et al., "Racial Variation in Serum Creatine Kinase Unrelated to Lean Body Mass," *Rheumatology* 29, no. 5 (1990): 371–73.

11. Jay S. Kaufman, Joanna Merckx, and Richard S. Cooper, "Use of Racial and Ethnic Categories in Medical Testing and Diagnosis: Primum Non Nocere," *Clinical Chemistry* 67, no. 11 (2021): 1456–65.

12. National Center for Health Statistics (NCHS), *National Health and Nutrition Examination Survey Data* (U.S. Department of Health and Human Services, Centers for Disease Control and Prevention, 2013–2014), https://wwwn.cdc.gov/nchs/nhanes/continuousnhanes/default.aspx?BeginYear=2013.

13. Zhong Cheng Luo, Kerstin Albertsson-Wikland, and Johan Karlberg, "Target Height as Predicted by Parental Heights in a Population-Based Study," *Pediatric Research* 44, no. 4 (1998): 563–71.

14. Michael W. Kattan, "Judging New Markers by Their Ability to Improve Predictive Accuracy," *Journal of the National Cancer Institute* 95, no. 9 (2003): 634–35.

15. Nwamaka D. Eneanya et al., "Health Inequities and the Inappropriate Use of Race in Nephrology," *Nature Reviews Nephrology* 18, no. 2 (2022): 84–94.

16. Juliana A. Zanocco et al., "Race Adjustment for Estimating Glomerular Filtration Rate Is Not Always Necessary," *Nephron* 2, no. 1 (2012): 293–302.

17. Cynthia Delgado et al., "Reassessing the Inclusion of Race in Diagnosing Kidney Diseases: An Interim Report from the NKF-ASN Task Force," *American Journal of Kidney Diseases* 78, no. 1 (2021): 103–15.

18. Jennifer W. Tsai et al., "Evaluating the Impact and Rationale of Race-Specific Estimations of Kidney Function: Estimations from US NHANES, 2015–2018," *EClinicalMedicine* 42 (2021): 101197.

19. Sam Zhang et al., "An Illusion of Predictability in Scientific Results: Even Experts Confuse Inferential Uncertainty and Outcome Variability," *Proceedings of the National Academy of Sciences* 120, no. 33 (2023): e2302491120.

20. U.S. Census, "Wealth Inequality in the U.S. by Household Type," August 1, 2022, https://www.census.gov/library/stories/2022/08/wealth-inequality-by-household-type.html.

21. Darshali A. Vyas, Leo G. Eisenstein, and David S. Jones, "Hidden in Plain Sight—Reconsidering the Use of Race Correction in Clinical Algorithms," *New England Journal of Medicine* 383, no. 9 (2020): 874–82.

22. Sonja B. Starr, "Race-Norming and Statistical Discrimination: Beyond the NFL," University of Chicago, Public Law Working Paper No. 805. Available at SSRN 4101693, 2022.

23. Tracie Canada and Chelsey R. Carter, "The NFL's Racist 'Race Norming' Is an Afterlife of Slavery," *Scientific American*, July 8, 2021, https://www.scientificamerican.com/article/the-nfls-racist-race-norming-is-an-afterlife-of-slavery/.

24. Katherine L. Possin, Elena Tsoy, and Charles C. Windon, "Perils of Race-Based Norms in Cognitive Testing: The Case of Former NFL Players," *JAMA Neurology* 78, no. 4 (2021): 377–78.

25. Jay S. Kaufman, "Ethical Dilemmas in Statistical Practice: The Problem of Race in Biomedicine," in *Mapping "Race": Critical Approaches to Health Disparities Research* (Rutgers University Press, 2013).

26. Sander Greenland, "Principles of Multilevel Modelling," *International Journal of Epidemiology* 29, no. 1 (2000): 158–67.

27. J. Martin Bland and Douglas G. Altman, "Statistics Notes: Some Examples of Regression Towards the Mean," *BMJ* 309, no. 6957 (1994): 780.

28. Bradley Efron and Carl Morris, "Stein's Paradox in Statistics," *Scientific American* 236, no. 5 (1977): 119–27.

29. Mayuri Mahendran, Daniel Lizotte, and Greta R. Bauer, "Describing Intersectional Health Outcomes: An Evaluation of Data Analysis Methods," *Epidemiology* 33, no. 3 (2022): 395.

30. Kimberly D. Acquaviva and Matthew Mintz, "Perspective: Are We Teaching Racial Profiling? The Dangers of Subjective Determinations of Race and Ethnicity in Case Presentations," *Academic Medicine* 85, no. 4 (2010): 702–5.

31. Ben Gose, "More Points for 'Strivers': The New Affirmative Action?," *Chronicle of Higher Education* 46, no. 4 (1999).

32. Nathan Glazer and A. Thernstrom, "Should the SAT Account for Race?," *New Republic* 221, no. 13 (1999): 26–29.

33. Amy Dockser Marcus, "To Spot Bias in SAT Questions, Test Maker Tests the Tests," *Wall Street Journal*, August 4, 1999, B1.

34. Howard Wainer, "Visual Revelations: Kelley's Paradox," *Chance* 13, no. 1 (2000): 47–48. This critique was published in 2000. In 2001, after twenty years at the Educational Testing Service, Howard Wainer left the company to take a position at the National Board of Medical Examiners (https://en.wikipedia.org/wiki/Howard_Wainer).

35. Howard Wainer and Lisa M. Brown, "Two Statistical Paradoxes in the Interpretation of Group Differences: Illustrated with Medical School Admission and Licensing Data," *American Statistician* 58, no. 2 (2004): 117–23.

36. Peter Schmidt, "ETS Accused of Squelching New Approach on Racial Bias," *Chronicle of Higher Education* 53, no. 12 (2006): A1–7.

37. Kaufman, "Ethical Dilemmas in Statistical Practice."

38. Alan M. Zaslavsky, "On Kelly's Paradox," *Chance* 13, no. 3 (2000): 3–4.

39. John Bailey Jones and Urvi Neelakantan, "A More Comprehensive Measure of the Black-White Wealth Gap," *Richmond Fed Economic Brief* 22, no. 17 (2022), https://www.richmondfed.org/publications/research/economic_brief/2022/eb_22-17.

40. Wikipedia, "List of U.S. States and Territories by African-American Population," https://en.wikipedia.org/wiki/List_of_U.S._states_and_territories_by_African-American_population;Wikipedia,"List of U.S. States and Territories by Income," https://en.wikipedia.org/wiki/List_of_U.S._states_and_territories_by_income.

41. Jason Gardosi et al., "Customized Growth Charts: Rationale, Validation and Clinical Benefits," *American Journal of Obstetrics and Gynecology* 218, no. 2 (2018): S609–18.

42. Marcelo L. Urquia, Howard Berger, and Joel G. Ray, "Risk of Adverse Outcomes Among Infants of Immigrant Women According to Birth-Weight Curves Tailored to Maternal World Region of Origin," *CMAJ* 187, no. 1 (2015): E32–40.

43. Germaine M. Buck Louis et al., "Racial/Ethnic Standards for Fetal Growth: The NICHD Fetal Growth Studies," *American Journal of Obstetrics and Gynecology* 213, no. 4 (2015): 449-e1.

44. José Villar et al., "The Likeness of Fetal Growth and Newborn Size Across Non-Isolated Populations in the INTERGROWTH-21st Project: The Fetal Growth Longitudinal Study and Newborn Cross-Sectional Study," *Lancet Diabetes and Endocrinology* 2, no. 10 (2014): 781–92.

45. Katherine L. Grantz et al., "Unified Standard for Fetal Growth: The Eunice Kennedy Shriver National Institute of Child Health and Human Development Fetal Growth Studies," *American Journal of Obstetrics and Gynecology* 226, no. 4 (2022): 576–87.

46. Rishi Caleyachetty et al., "Ethnicity-Specific BMI Cutoffs for Obesity Based on Type 2 Diabetes Risk in England: A Population-Based Cohort Study," *Lancet Diabetes and Endocrinology* 9, no. 7 (2021): 419–26.

47. Nitin Kapoor et al., "Normal Weight Obesity: An Underrecognized Problem in Individuals of South Asian Descent," *Clinical Therapeutics* 41, no. 8 (2019): 1638–42.

48. Michael G. Marmot and S. Leonard Syme, "Acculturation and Coronary Heart Disease in Japanese-Americans," *American Journal of Epidemiology* 104, no. 3 (1976): 225–47.

49. Marti Loring and Brian Powell, "Gender, Race, and DSM-III: A Study of the Objectivity of Psychiatric Diagnostic Behavior," *Journal of Health and Social Behavior* 29 (1988): 1–22.

50. Harold W. Neighbors et al., "The Influence of Racial Factors on Psychiatric Diagnosis: A Review and Suggestions for Research," *Community Mental Health Journal* 25 (1989): 301–11.

51. Amy L. Johnson, "Psychotic White Men and Bipolar Black Women? Racialized and Gendered Implications of Mental Health Terminology," *Social Science and Medicine* 352 (2024): 117015.

52. Jonathan Guryan and Kerwin Kofi Charles, "Taste-Based or Statistical Discrimination: The Economics of Discrimination Returns to Its Roots," *Economic Journal* 123, no. 572 (2013): F417–32.

53. J. Aislinn Bohren et al., "Inaccurate Statistical Discrimination: An Identification Problem," *Review of Economics and Statistics* (2023): 1–45, https://doi.org/10.1162/rest_a_01367.

54. Jessica K. Paulus and David M. Kent, "Predictably Unequal: Understanding and Addressing Concerns That Algorithmic Clinical Prediction May Increase Health Disparities," *NPJ Digital Medicine* 3, no. 1 (2020): 99.

55. Renée B. Adams et al., "Gendered Prices," *Review of Financial Studies* 34, no. 8 (2021): 3789–839.

56. Claudia Goldin and Cecilia Rouse, "Orchestrating Impartiality: The Impact of 'Blind' Auditions on Female Musicians," *American Economic Review* 90, no. 4 (2000): 715–41.

8. Filters and Screens

1. Ronald L. Wasserstein and Nicole A. Lazar, "The ASA Statement on P-Values: Context, Process, and Purpose," *American Statistician* 70, no. 2 (2016): 129–33.

2. Joseph L. Gastwirth, "Statistical Considerations Support the Supreme Court's Decision in *Matrixx Initiatives v. Siracusano*," *Jurimetrics* 52 (2011): 155.

3. Valentin Amrhein, Sander Greenland, and Blake McShane, "Scientists Rise Up Against Statistical Significance," *Nature* 567, no. 7748 (2019): 305–7.

4. This turns out to be not quite true, but it's close enough for our purposes. František Bartoš et al., "Fair Coins Tend to Land on the Same Side They Started: Evidence from 350,757 Flips," arXiv preprint arXiv:2310.04153 (2023).

5. Sander Greenland et al., "Statistical Tests, P Values, Confidence Intervals, and Power: A Guide to Misinterpretations," *European Journal of Epidemiology* 31 (2016): 337–50.

6. Andrew Gelman and Hal Stern, "The Difference Between 'Significant' and 'Not Significant' Is Not Itself Statistically Significant," *American Statistician* 60, no. 4 (2006): 328–31.

7. Alain Koyama et al., "Association Between the Mediterranean Diet and Cognitive Decline in a Biracial Population," *Journals of Gerontology Series A: Biomedical Sciences and Medical Sciences* 70, no. 3 (2015): 354–59.

8. ScienceDaily, "Mediterranean Diet Has Varied Effects on Cognitive Decline Among Different Races, Study Shows," July 16, 2014, https://www.sciencedaily.com/releases/2014/07/140716123843.htm.

9. The plot shows a Gaussian distribution for whites with a mean of 0.09 and standard deviation of 0.031 and a Gaussian distribution for Blacks with a mean of 0.22 and standard deviation of 0.087. These standard deviations are obtained by inverting the confidence intervals. For example, the white standard deviation is $(0.21 - (-0.03)) / (2 \times 1.96) = 0.12 / 3.92 = 0.031$, where -0.03 and 0.21

are the limits and 1.96 is the Z-score for the 97.5th percentile of the Guassian distribution. These are estimated density functions, and so the larger sample size of the white group is not depicted.

10. Jay S. Kaufman and Richard F. MacLehose, "Which of These Things Is Not Like the Others?," *Cancer* 119, no. 24 (2013): 4216–22.

11. Pieter Stijnen et al., "The Association of Common Variants in PCSK1 with Obesity: A HuGE Review and Meta-Analysis," *American Journal of Epidemiology* 180, no. 11 (2014): 1051–65.

12. Daniela Zanetti and Michael E. Weale, "Transethnic Differences in GWAS Signals: A Simulation Study," *Annals of Human Genetics* 82, no. 5 (2018): 280–86. Studies with larger numbers of Hispanics have revealed significant associations between the same rs6232 SNP in PCSK1 and obesity, for example, Marisela Villalobos-Comparan et al., "PCSK1 rs6232 Is Associated with Childhood and Adult Class III Obesity in the Mexican Population," *PloS One* 7, no. 6 (2012): e39037.

13. The probability of a straight is 0.0039 in a five-card hand, so calculating the probability of zero successes in one hundred trials using the binomial formula yields 68 percent, meaning that 32 percent of the time at least one flush will be observed among the one hundred hands.

14. P. C. Austin et al., "Testing Multiple Statistical Hypotheses Resulted in Spurious Associations: A Study of Astrological Signs and Health," *Journal of Clinical Epidemiology* 59, no. 9 (2006): 964–69. https://doi.org/10.1016/j.jclinepi.2006.01.012.

15. Lynn Eaton, "AIDS Vaccine May Offer Hope Only for Some Ethnic Groups," *BMJ* 326 (2003): 463.

16. $(4/203)/(9/111) = 0.24$, which is presumably the basis for the claim of a "76 percent reduction."

17. Mike Mitka, "Critics Bash HIV Vaccine Trial Analysis," *JAMA* 289, no. 12 (2003): 1491.

18. Sabin Russell and Tom Abate, "Scientists Split Over Role of Race in AIDS Vaccine/Struggle to Explain Whether Ethnicity Affected Results," *SF Gate*, February 25, 2003, https://www.sfgate.com/health/article/Scientists-split-over-role-of-race-in-AIDS-2632516.php.

19. Sander Greenland, "Randomization, Statistics, and Causal Inference," *Epidemiology* 1, no. 6 (1990): 421–29.

20. Jay S. Kaufman, Richard S. Cooper, and Daniel L. McGee, "Socioeconomic Status and Health in Blacks and Whites: The Problem of Residual Confounding and the Resiliency of Race," *Epidemiology* 8 (1997): 621–28.

21. Francesca Khani et al., "Evidence for Molecular Differences in Prostate Cancer Between African American and Caucasian Men," *Clinical Cancer Research* 20, no. 18 (2014): 4925–34.

22. Shiv K. Srivastava et al., "Genomic Rearrangements Associated with Prostate Cancer and Methods of Using the Same," https://patents.google.com/patent/WO2015103287A2/en.

23. Jay S. Kaufman and Richard S. Cooper, "In Search of the Hypothesis," *Public Health Reports* 110, no. 6 (1995): 662–66.

24. Lon R. Cardon and Lyle J. Palmer, "Population Stratification and Spurious Allelic Association," *Lancet* 361, no. 9357 (2003): 598–604.

25. E. S. Lander and N. J. Schork, "Genetic Dissection of Complex Traits," *Science* 265, no. 5181 (1994): 2037–48.

26. William C. Knowler et al., "Gm3; 5, 13, 14 and Type 2 Diabetes Mellitus: An Association in American Indians with Genetic Admixture," *American Journal of Human Genetics* 43, no. 4 (1988): 520.

27. Lynne C. Messer, J. Michael Oakes, and Susan Mason, "Effects of Socioeconomic and Racial Residential Segregation on Preterm Birth: A Cautionary Tale of Structural Confounding," *American Journal of Epidemiology* 171, no. 6 (2010): 664–73.

28. John P. A. Ioannidis, "Why Most Discovered True Associations Are Inflated," *Epidemiology* 19 (2008): 640–48.

29. Deirdre Nansen McCloskey and Steve Ziliak, *The Cult of Statistical Significance: How the Standard Error Costs Us Jobs, Justice, and Lives* (University of Michigan Press, 2010).

30. Greenland, "Randomization, Statistics, and Causal Inference."

31. For example, I have argued that, in the context of model selection, testing for the inclusion or exclusion of interaction terms to permit heterogeneous effect sizes is more defensible. This is because it really is about making a binary decision about differences being large or small with respect to sampling variability, which is exactly what significance tests assess. See Kaufman and MacLehose, "Which of These Things Is Not Like the Others?"

9. Scales, Values, and Preferences

1. WorldData, "Average Height and Weight by Country," April 2025, https://www.worlddata.info/average-bodyheight.php.

2. If you're wondering why a ratio of 2.5 is a 150 percent excess and not a 250 percent excess, it is important to remember that when two numbers are equal, the first is 0 percent larger than the second. If we then double the first number, it becomes 100 percent larger, which means that a ratio of 2 corresponds to a 100 percent excess and thus a ratio of 2.5 corresponds to a 150 percent excess. See Ashley H. Schempf and Jay S. Kaufman, "On the Percent of Excess Risk Explained," *Journal of Epidemiology and Community Health* 65, no. 2 (2011): 190.

3. Lisa M. Schwartz et al., "Ratio Measures in Leading Medical Journals: Structured Review of Accessibility of Underlying Absolute Risks," *BMJ* 333, no. 7581 (2006): 1248.

4. Ian N. Gregory, "Comparisons Between Geographies of Mortality and Deprivation from the 1900s and 2001: Spatial Analysis of Census and Mortality Statistics," *BMJ* 339 (2009): b3454.

5. Jennifer M. Orsi, Helen Margellos-Anast, and Steven Whitman, "Black–White Health Disparities in the United States and Chicago: A 15-Year Progress Analysis," *American Journal of Public Health* 100, no. 2 (2010): 349–56.

6. Sam Harper et al., "Implicit Value Judgments in the Measurement of Health Inequalities," *Milbank Quarterly* 88, no. 1 (2010): 4–29.

7. Allan Low and Anne Low, "Importance of Relative Measures in Policy on Health Inequalities," *BMJ* 332, no. 7547 (2006): 967–69.

8. Monica J. Alexander, Mathew V. Kiang, and Magali Barbieri, "Trends in Black and White Opioid Mortality in the United States, 1979–2015," *Epidemiology* 29, no. 5 (2018): 707–15.

9. Jay S. Kaufman, "Toward a More Disproportionate Epidemiology," *Epidemiology* 21, no. 1 (2010): 1–2.

10. Ashley I. Naimi and Brian W. Whitcomb, "Estimating Risk Ratios and Risk Differences Using Regression," *American Journal of Epidemiology* 189, no. 6 (2020): 508–10.

11. J. A. Tapia and F. J. Nieto, "Razón de Posibilidades: A Proposed Translation of the Term Odds Ratio," *Salud Publica de Mexico* 35, no. 4 (1993): 419–24.

12. Huw Talfryn Oakley Davies, Iain Kinloch Crombie, and Manouche Tavakoli, "When Can Odds Ratios Mislead?," *BMJ* 316, no. 7136 (1998): 989–91.

13. Kevin A. Schulman et al., "The Effect of Race and Sex on Physicians' Recommendations for Cardiac Catheterization," *New England Journal of Medicine* 340, no. 8 (1999): 618–26.

14. Lisa M. Schwartz, Steven Woloshin, and H. Gilbert Welch, "Misunderstandings About the Effects of Race and Sex on Physicians' Referrals for Cardiac Catheterization," *New England Journal of Medicine* 341, no. 4 (1999): 279–83.

15. R. Rubin, "Heart Care Reflects Race and Sex, Not Symptoms," *USA Today*, 1999. Cited in Schwartz et al., "Misunderstandings About the Effects of Race and Sex on Physicians' Referrals for Cardiac Catheterization."

16. Jay S. Kaufman, "Marginalia: Comparing Adjusted Effect Measures," *Epidemiology* 21, no. 4 (2010): 490–93.

17. Robin Gomila, "Logistic or Linear? Estimating Causal Effects of Experimental Treatments on Binary Outcomes Using Regression Analysis," *Journal of Experimental Psychology: General* 150, no. 4 (2021): 700.

18. Richard J. Cook and David L. Sackett, "The Number Needed to Treat: A Clinically Useful Measure of Treatment Effect," *BMJ* 310, no. 6977 (1995): 452–54.

19. Stacey Jolly et al., "Higher Cardiovascular Disease Prevalence and Mortality Among Younger Blacks Compared to Whites," *American Journal of Medicine* 123, no. 9 (2010): 811–18.

20. Jay S. Kaufman, Sam Harper, and Nicholas B. King, "A More Complete Picture of Higher Cardiovascular Disease Prevalence Among Blacks Compared to Whites," *American Journal of Medicine* 124, no. 5 (2011): e5–e6.

21. Joseph B. Kadane, "Odds Ratios as a Measure of Disproportionate Treatment: Application to Jury Venires," *Law, Probability and Risk* 21, no. 3–4 (2022): 163–73.

22. Where S = being stopped, B = being Black, and ~B = not being Black, then

1. $P(S|B) = P(S \& B)/P(B) = P(B|S)P(S)/P(B)$
2. $P(S|{\sim}B) = P({\sim}B|S)P(S)/P(B)$

The ratio of these two expressions = $P(S|B)/P(S|{\sim}B)$ is the intuitive comparison of interest for the judge. When expression 1 is divided by expression 2, the P(S) terms cancel out, leaving $[P(B|S)/P(B)]/[P({\sim}B|S)/P({\sim}B)$, which can be rearranged to yield $[P(B|S)/P({\sim}B|S)] \times [P({\sim}B)/P(B)]$, which is the odds of being Black if stopped divided by the odds of being Black. Stated this way, the odds ratio would be difficult for a judge or jury to understand, but restating it as the numerically equivalent proportion stopped among Blacks versus non-Blacks becomes very intuitive. This follows from the comparison against the whole population, which might be more common in a legal context than in a biomedical context.

23. James P. Scanlan, "Guest Editorial: Can We Actually Measure Health Disparities?," *Chance* 19, no. 2 (2006): 47–51.

24. "Homeopathic paradox" is my term not Scanlan's. I am referring to a central tenet of homeopathic medicine, which is homeopathic dilution. This is the process of making a medicine by repeatedly diluting a solution until there is less than one molecule remaining of the curative substance, only the memory of that substance in the diluent. The power of the cure is purportedly maximized at the moment that it completely disappears.

25. James P. Scanlan, "The Mismeasure of Health Disparities," *Journal of Public Health Management and Practice* 22, no. 4 (2016): 415–19.

26. Frank Cowell, *Measuring Inequality* (Oxford University Press, 2011).

10. What Explains a Disparity?

1. There are many textbooks on this topic, including Tyler VanderWeele, *Explanation in Causal Inference: Methods for Mediation and Interaction* (Oxford University Press, 2015); and David P. MacKinnon, *Introduction to Statistical Mediation Analysis* (Routledge, 2012).

2. Enrique F. Schisterman, Stephen R. Cole, and Robert W. Platt, "Overadjustment Bias and Unnecessary Adjustment in Epidemiologic Studies," *Epidemiology* 20, no. 4 (2009): 488–95.

3. James M. Robins and Sander Greenland, "Identifiability and Exchangeability for Direct and Indirect Effects," *Epidemiology* 3, no. 2 (1992): 143–55.

4. Robins and Greenland, "Identifiability and Exchangeability for Direct and Indirect Effects."

5. Judea Pearl, "Direct and Indirect Effects," in *Probabilistic and Causal Inference: The Works of Judea Pearl* (Association for Computing Machinery, 2022).

6. Tyler J. VanderWeele and Whitney R. Robinson, "On Causal Interpretation of Race in Regressions Adjusting for Confounding and Mediating Variables," *Epidemiology* 25, no. 4 (2014): 473–84.

7. Of course we can also condition on other covariates, for example taking a random income from a person with the same level of attained education.

8. Nancy Krieger, "On the Causal Interpretation of Race [Letter]," *Epidemiology* 25 (2014): 937

9. Frederick L. Brancati et al., "The Excess Incidence of Diabetic End-Stage Renal Disease Among Blacks: A Population-Based Study of Potential Explanatory Factors," *JAMA* 268, no. 21 (1992): 3079–84.

10. Brancati et al., "The Excess Incidence of Diabetic End-Stage Renal Disease Among Blacks," 3084.

11. RationalWiki, "Holmesian Fallacy," February 8, 2025, https://rationalwiki.org/wiki/Holmesian_fallacy.

12. Jay S. Kaufman, Richard S. Cooper, and Daniel L. McGee, "Socioeconomic Status and Health in Blacks and Whites: The Problem of Residual Confounding and the Resiliency of Race," *Epidemiology* 8 (1997): 621–28.

13. Tyler J. VanderWeele, Linda Valeri, and Elizabeth L. Ogburn, "The Role of Measurement Error and Misclassification in Mediation Analysis," *Epidemiology* 23, no. 4 (2012): 561–64.

14. Ezra Klein, "The Sam Harris Debate," Vox, April 9, 2018, https://www.vox.com/2018/4/9/17210248/sam-harris-ezra-klein-charles-murray-transcript-podcast.

15. Richard J. Herrnstein and Charles Murray, *The Bell Curve: Intelligence and Class Structure in American Life* (Simon and Schuster, 1994).

16. Bernie Devlin et al., *Intelligence, Genes, and Success: Scientists Respond to* The Bell Curve (Springer, 1997).

17. Melissa Bartick et al., "The Role of Breastfeeding in Racial and Ethnic Disparities in Sudden Unexpected Infant Death: A Population-Based Study of 13 Million Infants in the United States," *American Journal of Epidemiology* 191, no. 7 (2022): 1190–201.

18. Patricia J. Martens, "What Do Kramer's Baby-Friendly Hospital Initiative PRO-BIT Studies Tell Us? A Review of a Decade of Research," *Journal of Human Lactation* 28, no. 3 (2012): 335–42.

19. Graham Dunn, "Complier-Average Causal Effect (CACE) Estimation," in *International Encyclopedia of Statistical Science* (Springer, 2011).

20. Ashley I. Naimi, Jay S. Kaufman, and Richard F. MacLehose, "Mediation Misgivings: Ambiguous Clinical and Public Health Interpretations of Natural Direct and Indirect Effects," *International Journal of Epidemiology* 43, no. 5 (2014): 1656–61.

21. This is referred to as the "Baron and Kenny Approach," after a seminal article: Reuben M. Baron and David A. Kenny, "The Moderator–Mediator Variable Distinction in Social Psychological Research: Conceptual, Strategic, and Statistical Considerations," *Journal of Personality and Social Psychology* 51, no. 6 (1986): 1173–82. With over 130,000 citations, this is one of the most highly referenced papers in all of social science.

22. E. Cuyler Hammond, Irving J. Selikoff, and Herbert Seidman, "Asbestos Exposure, Cigarette Smoking and Death Rates," *Annals of the New York Academy of Sciences* 330, no. 1 (1979): 473–790.

23. Jay S. Kaufman, Richard F. MacLehose, and Sol Kaufman, "A Further Critique of the Analytic Strategy of Adjusting for Covariates to Identify Biologic Mediation," *Epidemiologic Perspectives and Innovations* 1 (2004): 4.

24. Mayuri Mahendran, Daniel Lizotte, and Greta R. Bauer, "Describing Intersectional Health Outcomes: An Evaluation of Data Analysis Methods," *Epidemiology* 33, no. 3 (2022): 395–405.

25. James C. Barnes and Ryan T. Motz, "Reducing Racial Inequalities in Adulthood Arrest by Reducing Inequalities in School Discipline: Evidence from the School-to-Prison Pipeline," *Developmental Psychology* 54, no. 12 (2018): 2328.

26. Astute readers may note that the Black and white adjusted risks of suspension/expulsion are both lower than the average risk of 25.3 percent cited earlier. This is because the adjustments are to the overall distribution of covariates, which is dominated by the white students who make up 76.5 percent of the sample. Therefore, the adjusted risks for Black students reflect those under social and economic circumstances that are more advantaged than they actually experience, which is another reminder of how tricky adjustments can be if they are not interpreted critically.

27. It is also problematic in this context to use the odds ratio because the outcome is not rare. The authors acknowledge this limitation.

28. For an example of a racial/ethnic disparities article in which this is done correctly, see for example Katrina L. Devick et al., "The Role of Body Mass Index at Diagnosis of Colorectal Cancer on Black–White Disparities in Survival: A Density Regression Mediation Approach," *Biostatistics* 23, no. 2 (2022): 449–66. The highly technical nature of this paper demonstrates that proper handling of the mediational analysis in this setting is not a simple task.

29. Erica L. Green and Katie Benner, "Trump Parkland Inquiry Attacks Protections for Minority Students," *New York Times*, December 17, 2018, Section A, Page 1, https://www.nytimes.com/2018/12/17/us/politics/trump-school-discipline

.html; Lauren Camera, "The Race Research Cited by DeVos," *US News and World Report*, March 28, 2019, https://www.usnews.com/news/education-news /articles/2019-03-28/the-controversial-race-research-devos-used-to-revoke-school -discipline-guidance.

30. Richard O. Welsh, "Up the Down Escalator? Examining a Decade of School Discipline Reforms," *Children and Youth Services Review* 150 (2023): 106962.

31. Jay S. Kaufman, "Statistics, Adjusted Statistics, and Maladjusted Statistics," *American Journal of Law and Medicine* 43, no. 2–3 (2017): 193–208.

32. Sharmilee M. Nyenhuis et al., "Race Is Associated with Differences in Airway Inflammation in Patients with Asthma," *Journal of Allergy and Clinical Immunology* 140, no. 1 (2017): 257–65.

33. Torie Grant, Emily Croce, and Elizabeth C. Matsui, "Asthma and the Social Determinants of Health," *Annals of Allergy, Asthma and Immunology* 128, no. 1 (2022): 5–11.

34. Nyenhuis et al., "Race Is Associated with Differences in Airway Inflammation in Patients with Asthma." Quote was taken from the article abstract.

35. Douglas C. Cowan et al., "Effects of Steroid Therapy on Inflammatory Cell Subtypes in Asthma," *Thorax* 65, no. 5 (2010): 384–90.

36. University of Illinois at Chicago, "Why Is Asthma Worse in Black Patients?," Science-Daily, January 6, 2017, www.sciencedaily.com/releases/2017/01/170106133056. htm.

11. Nature Versus Nurture

1. National Institute for Health and Care Excellence, "Hypertension in Adults: Diagnosis and Management," August 28, 2019, https://www.nice.org.uk/guidance /ng136/chapter/Recommendations#starting-antihypertensive-drug-treatment.

2. Kenneth E. Bernstein et al., "A Modern Understanding of the Traditional and Nontraditional Biological Functions of Angiotensin-Converting Enzyme," *Pharmacological Reviews* 65, no. 1 (2013): 1–46.

3. Paul A. James et al., "2014 Evidence-Based Guideline for the Management of High Blood Pressure in Adults: Report from the Panel Members Appointed to the Eighth Joint National Committee (JNC 8)," *JAMA* 311, no. 5 (2014): 507–20.

4. The term "black" is not capitalized in the published Joint National Committee report (2014), although it is published in *JAMA*, which now routinely capitalizes the term "Black" when it is used to designate race. See Annette Flanagin et al., "Updated Guidance on the Reporting of Race and Ethnicity in Medical and Science Journals," *JAMA* 326, no. 7 (2021): 621–27.

5. Andrea Westby, Ebiere Okah, and Jason Ricco, "Race-Based Treatment Decisions Perpetuate Structural Racism," *American Family Physician* 102, no. 3 (2020): 136–37.

6. Jackson T. Wright et al., "Outcomes in Hypertensive Black and Nonblack Patients Treated with Chlorthalidone, Amlodipine, and Lisinopril," *JAMA* 293, no. 13 (2005): 1595–608.

7. There are two values measured for blood pressure: the systolic blood pressure, which is the maximum pressure obtained when the heart contracts, and the diastolic blood pressure, which is the minimum pressure to which it falls between heartbeats. To keep things concise, when I refer to "blood pressure" in this chapter, I am referring only to the systolic pressure.

8. Jay S. Kaufman and Richard S. Cooper, "Use of Racial and Ethnic Identity in Medical Evaluations and Treatments," in *What's the Use of Race? Modern Governance and the Biology of Difference*, ed. Ian Whitmarsh and David S. Jones (MIT Press, 2010).

9. A subsequent 2013 meta-analysis included a few more studies and came to roughly the same estimate of just over 4 millimeters of mercury difference between the response of whites and Blacks: Robert N. Peck et al., "Difference in Blood Pressure Response to ACE-Inhibitor Monotherapy Between Black and White Adults with Arterial Hypertension: A Meta-Analysis of 13 Clinical Trials," *BMC Nephrology* 14 (2013): 1–11.

10. Ashwini R. Sehgal, "Overlap Between Whites and Blacks in Response to Antihypertensive Drugs," *Hypertension* 43, no. 3 (2004): 566–72.

11. Margaret Sullivan Pepe et al., "Limitations of the Odds Ratio in Gauging the Performance of a Diagnostic, Prognostic, or Screening Marker," *American Journal of Epidemiology* 159, no. 9 (2004): 882–90.

12. N. J. Wald, A. K. Hackshaw, and C. D. Frost, "When Can a Risk Factor Be Used as a Worthwhile Screening Test?," *BMJ* 319, no. 7224 (1999): 1562–65.

13. Charles F. Manski, John Mullahy, and Atheendar S. Venkataramani, "Using Measures of Race to Make Clinical Predictions: Decision Making, Patient Health, and Fairness," *Proceedings of the National Academy of Sciences* 120, no. 35 (2023): e2303370120.

14. Dipesh P. Gopal and Rohin Francis, "Does Race Belong in the Hypertension Guidelines?," *Journal of Human Hypertension* 35, no. 10 (2021): 940–41.

15. Jash S. Parikh et al., "The Association Between Antihypertensive Medication Use and Blood Pressure Is Influenced by Obesity," *Journal of Obesity* 1 (2018): 4573258.

16. Another issue is dosage. Peck and colleagues showed that the Black-white difference in treatment response could be reduced if Blacks were simply given a higher dose of angiotensin-converting enzyme inhibitors. Peck et al., "Difference in Blood Pressure Response to ACE-Inhibitor Monotherapy Between Black and White Adults with Arterial Hypertension." Dosage is not generally assigned per body weight, for example, and Blacks may also present with more severe hypertension on average; Richard S. Cooper, Youlian Liao, and Charles Rotimi, "Is Hypertension

More Severe Among US Blacks, or Is Severe Hypertension More Common?," *Annals of Epidemiology* 6, no. 3 (1996): 173–80.

17. Jay S. Kaufman and Susan A. Hall, "The Slavery Hypertension Hypothesis: Dissemination and Appeal of a Modern Race Theory," *Epidemiology* 14, no. 1 (2003): 111–18.

18. Richard S. Cooper et al., "An International Comparative Study of Blood Pressure in Populations of European vs. African Descent," *BMC Medicine* 3 (2005): 1–8.

19. Richard Cooper and Charles Rotimi, "Hypertension in Populations of West African Origin: Is There a Genetic Predisposition?," *Journal of Hypertension* 12, no. 3 (1994): 215–28; Stephen G. Rostand, "Ultraviolet Light May Contribute to Geographic and Racial Blood Pressure Differences," *Hypertension* 30, no. 2 (1997): 150–56; Lee Ellis and Helmuth Nyborg, "Racial/Ethnic Variations in Male Testosterone Levels: A Probable Contributor to Group Differences in Health," *Steroids* 57, no. 2 (1992): 72–75.

20. Thomas W. Wilson and Clarence E. Grim, "Biohistory of Slavery and Blood Pressure Differences in Blacks Today: A Hypothesis," *Hypertension* 17, no. 1 (1991): I122.

21. Jared J. Diamond, "The Salt-Shaker's Curse," *Natural History* 10 (1991): 20–26. Diamond begins by posing the question, "What is it about American blacks that makes them disproportionately likely to develop hypertension and then to die of its consequences?"

22. Richard S. Cooper and Xiaofeng Zhu, "Racial Differences and the Genetics of Hypertension," *Current Hypertension Reports* 3, no. 1 (2001): 19–24.

23. George B. J. Busby et al., "Admixture into and Within Sub-Saharan Africa," *eLife* 5 (2016): e15266.

24. Ann Gibbons, "Shedding Light on Skin Color," *Science* 346, no. 6212 (2014): 934–36.

25. Nina G. Jablonski and George Chaplin, "The Colours of Humanity: The Evolution of Pigmentation in the Human Lineage," *Philosophical Transactions of the Royal Society B: Biological Sciences* 372, no. 1724 (2017): 20160349.

26. Heather L. Norton et al., "Genetic Evidence for the Convergent Evolution of Light Skin in Europeans and East Asians," *Molecular Biology and Evolution* 24, no. 3 (2007): 710–22.

27. Dirk Schadendorf et al., "Melanoma," *Lancet* 392, no. 10151 (2018): 971–84.

28. Note that the E × G product will be 0 when either E = 0 or G = 0 because anything multiplied by 0 equals 0. This means that the β_3 term only contributes something in the E = 1 and G = 1 situation, which refers to dark skin in high ultraviolet (UV) light. The value of the β_3 term will be negative to conform to the expectation that ill health is reduced by this combination of exposures.

29. By canceling out terms when they are multiplied by 0, one can derive from this regression equation that the expected average value of Y under each of the four conditions is as follows:

Light skin (G = 0), low UV radiation (E = 0): Average Y = β_0
Light skin (G = 0), high UV radiation (E = 1): Average Y = $\beta_0 + \beta_1$
Dark skin (G = 1), low UV radiation (E = 0): Average Y = $\beta_0 + \beta_2$
Dark skin (G = 1), high UV radiation (E = 1): Average Y = $\beta_0 + \beta_1 + \beta_2 + \beta_3$

30. Shaohua Fan et al., "Going Global by Adapting Local: A Review of Recent Human Adaptation," *Science* 354, no. 6308 (2016): 54–59.
31. Stephen M. Downes and Eric Turkheimer, "An Early History of the Heritability Coefficient Applied to Humans (1918–1960)," *Biological Theory* 17 (2021): 1–12.
32. Lucas J. Matthews and Eric Turkheimer, "Three Legs of the Missing Heritability Problem," *Studies in History and Philosophy of Science* 93 (2022): 183–91.
33. Jay Joseph, *The Missing Gene: Psychiatry, Heredity, and the Fruitless Search for Genes* (Algora, 2006), 34–36.
34. K. J. Rothman, *Epidemiology: An Introduction*, 2nd ed. (Oxford University Press, 2012), 25.
35. Or Zuk et al., "The Mystery of Missing Heritability: Genetic Interactions Create Phantom Heritability," *Proceedings of the National Academy of Sciences* 109, no. 4 (2012): 1193–98.
36. Erik Corona et al., "Analysis of the Genetic Basis of Disease in the Context of Worldwide Human Relationships and Migration," *PLoS Genetics* 9, no. 5 (2013): e1003447.
37. Stanford University Medical Center, "Diabetes' Genetic Underpinnings Can Vary Based on Ethnic Background," ScienceDaily, May 23, 2013, https://www.sciencedaily.com/releases/2013/05/130523162248.htm.
38. Richard S. Cooper and Jay S. Kaufman, "What Is the Relevance of Genetic Speculation That Contradicts Observed Reality?," Posted by jkaufman1 on May 28, 2013, at 19:29 GMT, https://journals.plos.org/plosgenetics/article/comment?id=10.1371/annotation/5dcab322-d620-4f9e-bfb0-6383bd42be9d.
39. Erik Corona, "RE: What Is the Relevance of Genetic Speculation That Contradicts Observed Reality?," ecoronap replied to jkaufman1 on July 6, 2013, at 13:22 GMT, https://journals.plos.org/plosgenetics/article/comment?id=10.1371/annotation/5dcab322-d620-4f9e-bfb0-6383bd42be9d.
40. Massimo Pigliucci and Maarten Boudry, eds., *Philosophy of Pseudoscience: Reconsidering the Demarcation Problem* (University of Chicago Press, 2019).
41. Christopher Jencks, *Inequality: A Reassessment of the Effect of Family and Schooling in America* (Basic Books, 1972).

42. Richard Cooper, "A Note on the Biologic Concept of Race and Its Application in Epidemiologic Research," *American Heart Journal* 108, no. 3 (1984): 715–23.

43. James Woodward and Kenneth Kendler, "Polygene Risk Scores: A Philosophical Exploration," *Philosophy of Medicine* 4, no. 1 (2023): 1–21.

44. Hans Fredrik Sunde et al., "Genetic Similarity Between Relatives Provides Evidence on the Presence and History of Assortative Mating," *Nature Communications* 15, no. 1 (2024): 2641.

45. W. Carson Byrd and Victor E. Ray, "Ultimate Attribution in the Genetic Era: White Support for Genetic Explanations of Racial Difference and Policies," *Annals of the American Academy of Political and Social Science* 661, no. 1 (2015): 212–35.

46. Keith Wailoo, *How Cancer Crossed the Color Line* (Oxford University Press, 2011). Wailoo cites the cancer surgeon Willy Meyer having noted in the early 1930s that primitive nonwhite people were not only immune from cancer "on par with the fish of the ocean" but also incapable of being aware of cancer even if they had it (5).

47. Santosh K. Singh, James W. Lillard Jr., and Rajesh Singh, "Molecular Basis for Prostate Cancer Racial Disparities," *Frontiers in Bioscience* 22 (2017): 428.

48. Patrick D. Evans et al., "Microcephalin, a Gene Regulating Brain Size, Continues to Evolve Adaptively in Humans," *Science* 309, no. 5741 (2005): 1717–20. See lengthy critique and discussion in Angela Saini, *Superior: The Return of Race Science* (Beacon, 2019).

49. Bob Holmes, "The Real First Farmers: How Agriculture Was a Global Invention," *New Scientist* 28 (2015), https://www.newscientist.com/article/mg22830450-700 -the-real-first-farmers-how-agriculture-was-a-global-invention/; and William G. Boltz, "Early Chinese Writing," *World Archaeology* 17, no. 3 (1986): 420–36.

50. Kevin M. Beaver et al., "Monoamine Oxidase A Genotype Is Associated with Gang Membership and Weapon Use," *Comprehensive Psychiatry* 51, no. 2 (2010): 130–34.

51. Kevin M. Beaver and Nicholas Chaviano, "The Association Between Genetic Risk and Contact with the Criminal Justice System in a Sample of Hispanics," *Journal of Contemporary Criminal Justice* 27, no. 1 (2011): 81–94.

52. Quamrul Ashraf and Oded Galor, "The 'Out of Africa' Hypothesis, Human Genetic Diversity, and Comparative Economic Development," *American Economic Review* 103, no. 1 (2013): 1–46.

53. Richard Lynn, "Reflections on Sixty-Eight Years of Research on Race and Intelligence," *Psych* 1, no. 1 (2019): 123–31.

54. Richard J. Herrnstein and Charles Murray, *The Bell Curve: Intelligence and Class Structure in American Life* (Free Press, 1994).

55. James J. Heckman, "Lessons from the Bell Curve," *Journal of Political Economy* 103, no. 5 (1995): 1113–14.

56. Bionity, "The Bell Curve," https://www.bionity.com/en/encyclopedia/The_ Bell_Curve.html.

57. Marcus R. Munafò et al., "A Manifesto for Reproducible Science," *Nature Human Behaviour* 1, no. 0021 (2017): 1–9.

58. Dara G. Torgerson et al., "Meta-Analysis of Genome-Wide Association Studies of Asthma in Ethnically Diverse North American Populations," *Nature Genetics* 43, no. 9 (2011): 887.

59. Recall that an allele is a specific location on the genome where the DNA sequence varies from person to person. When the code differs by a single one of the four DNA nucleotides, commonly abbreviated as A, G, T, or C, it is referred to as a SNP (pronounced "snip"), which stands for single nucleotide polymorphism. The human genome has about 3.2 billion loci (nucleotide pairs), of which 99.6 percent are identical in all people, leaving about 12 million places (0.4 percent) where the nucleotide at that location differs from one person to the next. Rachel Crowley, "Genetics by the Numbers," April 24, 2024, https://biobeat.nigms.nih.gov/2024/04/genetics-by-the-numbers/.

60. Julie Steenhuysen, "Gene Discovered That Raises Asthma Risk in Blacks," Reuters, July 31, 2011, https://www.reuters.com/article/us-asthma-genes-idUSTRE76U23I20110731.

61. Steenhuysen, "Gene Discovered That Raises Asthma Risk in Blacks."

62. David B. Kantor et al., "Replication and Fine Mapping of Asthma-Associated Loci in Individuals of African Ancestry," *Human Genetics* 132 (2013): 1039–47.

63. Matthew J. Page et al., "Investigating and Dealing with Publication Bias and Other Reporting Biases in Meta-Analyses of Health Research: A Review," *Research Synthesis Methods* 12, no. 2 (2021): 248–59.

64. Michelle Daya and Kathleen C. Barnes, "African American Ancestry Contribution to Asthma and Atopic Dermatitis," *Annals of Allergy, Asthma and Immunology* 122, no. 5 (2019): 456–62.

65. Tania M. Bubela and Timothy A. Caulfield, "Do the Print Media 'Hype' Genetic Research? A Comparison of Newspaper Stories and Peer-Reviewed Research Papers," *Canadian Medical Association Journal* 170, no. 9 (2004): 1399–407.

Conclusion

1. Lauren Davenport, "The Fluidity of Racial Classifications," *Annual Review of Political Science* 23, no. 1 (2020): 221–40.

2. Shira Mitchell et al., "Algorithmic Fairness: Choices, Assumptions, and Definitions," *Annual Review of Statistics and Its Application* 8, no. 1 (2021): 141–63.

3. Coleman Hughes, *The End of Race Politics: Arguments for a Colorblind America* (Thesis, 2024).

4. Kim Parker et al., "Race and Multiracial Americans in the US Census," Pew Research Center, Washington, DC, June 2015, https://www.pewresearch.org

/social-trends/2015/06/11/chapter-1-race-and-multiracial-americans-in-the-u
-s-census/.

5. Brittany Rico, Paul Jacobs, and Alli Coritz, "2020 Census Shows Increase in
Multiracial Population in All Age Categories," U.S. Census Bureau, June 1, 2023,
https://www.census.gov/library/stories/2023/06/nearly-a-third-reporting-two-or
-more-races-under-18-in-2020.html.

6. David E. Bernstein, *Classified: The Untold Story of Racial Classification in America*
(Bombardier, 2022), 110–12.

7. K. S. Joseph et al., "Temporal Changes in Maternal Mortality in the United
States," *American Journal of Obstetrics and Gynecology* 231 (2024): S0002-9378.

8. D. L. Hoyert, "Maternal Mortality Rates in the United States, 2021. NCHS Health
E-Stats. Centers for Disease Control and Prevention (CDC)," National Center for Health Statistics, 2023, https://www.cdc.gov/nchs/data/hestat/maternal
-mortality/2021/maternal-mortality-rates-2021.htm.

9. Michelle J. K. Osterman et al., "Births: Final Data for 2021," 2023, https://stacks
.cdc.gov/view/cdc/122047.

10. John W. Jackson et al., "Evaluating Effects of Multilevel Interventions on Disparity in Health and Healthcare Decisions," *Prevention Science* 25, suppl. 3 (2024):
407–20.

11. William G. Cochran, "Analysis of Covariance: Its Nature and Uses," *Biometrics* 13,
no. 3 (1957): 261–81.

12. Andrew Gelman and Eric Loken, "The Statistical Crisis in Science," *American
Scientist* 102, no. 6 (2014): 460–65.

13. Joel Best, *Damned Lies and Statistics: Untangling Numbers from the Media, Politicians,
and Activists* (University of California Press, 2012).

14. George E. P. Box, "Science and Statistics," *Journal of the American Statistical Association* 71, no. 356 (1976): 791–99.

15. Jennifer W. Tsai et al., "Evaluating the Impact and Rationale of Race-Specific
Estimations of Kidney Function: Estimations from US NHANES, 2015–2018,"
EClinicalMedicine 42 (2021): 101197.

16. Francis Fukuyama, *Identity: The Demand for Dignity and the Politics of Resentment*
(Farrar, Straus and Giroux, 2018).

17. Thomas Chatterton Williams, *Self-Portrait in Black and White: Unlearning Race*
(Hachette, 2019).

18. The term "sensitivity analyses" refers to a set of alternate specifications of the
model in which some aspects are varied to test their impact. For example, if I have
adjusted for covariate Z in my main model, then I may want to check the result
of another model that is the same except without the adjustment for Z. If the
results are sensitive to this change, then I had better be sure that I want to adjust
for Z because that decision is consequential. If, however, the result is roughly the
same either way, then the result is not sensitive to that choice and I don't have to

worry about it so much. Modeling requires many decisions along the way, and each can be subjected to this kind of sensitivity analysis to find out which decisions have a big impact on the final result and therefore require stronger justification. For example, Paul R. Rosenbaum, "Sensitivity Analysis in Observational Studies," *Encyclopedia of Statistics in Behavioral Science* 4 (2005): 1809–14.

19. Sander Greenland, "Randomization, Statistics, and Causal Inference," *Epidemiology* 1, no. 6 (1990): 421–29.
20. Valentin Amrhein, Sander Greenland, and Blake McShane, "Scientists Rise Up Against Statistical Significance," *Nature* 567, no. 7748 (2019): 305–7.
21. Clare R. Evans et al., "A Tutorial for Conducting Intersectional Multilevel Analysis of Individual Heterogeneity and Discriminatory Accuracy (MAIHDA)," *SSM-Population Health* 26 (2024): 101664.
22. Ting-Hsuan Chang, Trang Quynh Nguyen, and John W. Jackson, "The Importance of Equity Value Judgments and Estimator-Estimand Alignment in Measuring Disparity and Identifying Targets to Reduce Disparity," *American Journal of Epidemiology* 193, no. 3 (2024): 536–47.
23. L. Paloma Rojas-Saunero et al., "Racial and Ethnic Differences in the Risk of Dementia Diagnosis Under Hypothetical Blood Pressure–Lowering Interventions: The Multi-Ethnic Study of Atherosclerosis," *Alzheimer's and Dementia* 20, no. 8 (2024): 5271–80.
24. Paul Muntner et al., "Trends in Blood Pressure Control Among US Adults with Hypertension, 1999–2000 to 2017–2018," *JAMA* 324, no. 12 (2020): 1190–200.
25. Jay S. Kaufman, "Commentary: Causal Inference for Social Exposures," *Annual Review of Public Health* 40, no. 1 (2019): 7–21.
26. Roch A. Nianogo et al., "Medicaid Expansion and Racial–Ethnic and Sex Disparities in Cardiovascular Diseases Over 6 Years: A Generalized Synthetic Control Approach," *Epidemiology* 35, no. 2 (2024): 263–72.
27. Judea Pearl and Dana Mackenzie, *The Book of Why: The New Science of Cause and Effect* (Basic Books, 2018).
28. Charmont Wang, *Sense and Nonsense of Statistical Inference: Controversy: Misuse, and Subtlety* (CRC, 2020).
29. Inmaculada de Melo-Martin and Kristen K. Intemann, "Can Ethical Reasoning Contribute to Better Epidemiology? A Case Study in Research on Racial Health Disparities," *European Journal of Epidemiology* 22 (2007): 215–21.

Index

absolute contrasts, relative contrasts compared with, 144

absolute excess risk, 134

academic test performance, of schoolchildren, 106

ACE. *See* angiotensin-converting enzyme inhibitors

Adams, Renée, 114

Add Health. *See* National Longitudinal Study of Adolescent to Adult Health

adjusted disparities, crude disparities contrasted with, 46

adjusted effect estimates, sampling distributions and, *121*

adjusted estimate, randomized trial verifying, 37

adjusted models, equity judgments corresponding with, 50

adjusted rates, 38

adjusted results, crude results contrasted with, 189

adjusted scores, crude scores contrasted with, 53, *54*

adjustments, 18, 20, 36, 45–47, 55, 98–99, 221n26; age, 202n3; confounder, 150; to covariates, 52; for education, 126; effects estimated by, 163–64; for income, 126; inequality obscured by, 61; for mobility and risk, 56; to racial and ethnic disparities, 39–40, 187; racial disparities and, 153–54; real world contrasted with, 37; statistical

models for, 16–17. *See also* statistical adjustments

adjustment strategies, 4–5, 64

age, 103–4; cardiovascular disease mortality by race and, 40, *41*; COVID-19 vaccination and severe illness and, *22, 23, 24, 34,* 63, *64*; maternal mortality and race and, 185–86; racial and ethnic differences in mortality and, 76–77, *78*; racial differences in COVID-19 mortality confounded by, 53; stratified analysis confounded by, 23

age adjustment, 202n3

age distribution, 35–36

age pattern, in racial inequality, 144

age standardization, 42–45

age standards, racial and ethnic disparities and, 40

AIDSVAX, 124–25

algorithmic bias, 113

ALLHAT (trial), 167–69

Alzheimer's disease, smoking and, 76, 80

American College of Surgeons, 4

American Journal of Epidemiology, 155

American Journal of Public Health, 132

American Society of Nephrology, 103

American Statistical Association (ASA), 115

analysis: causal mediation, 161; critique of, 5; statistical, 16–17; stratified, 23

analysts, ethical responsibilities of, 190–91

ancestry, genetic, 85–86
ancestry estimation, 11–12
ancestry kits, commercial, 13–14
ancestry proportions, from DNA, 88
ancestry testing, 89–90
angiotensin-converting enzyme inhibitors
    (ACE), 167–68; dosage of, 223n16; systolic
    blood pressure and race and, *170*
Anglo names, 135, *136*, *137*
annual base salaries, 103
antimalarial drugs, randomized trials of, 202n2
Arab Americans, 85
arrests, student suspension or expulsion and
    race and, *161*, *162*
art auctions, 114
ASA. *See* American Statistical Association
asbestos, lung cancer and smoking and, 158
"Asian American," 84–85
association, as causation, 37
asthma, 164, 179–81
athletic ability, height not correlated with,
    64, *65*
Atlantic slave trade, 1
audit studies, 26–28, 140

bank loans, racial disparities in, 29–30
Barnes, James, 160, 162
Bartick, Melissa, 155, 157
Batenburg, Ann, 201n14
Battle of Hastings, 88
Beavis, Anna, 58, 60, 61
Bell Curve, The (Herrnstein and Murray), 155
Bernstein, David, 90
Bertrand, Marianne, 26
bias, 105, 149–50; algorithmic, 113; in causal
    estimations, 27; clinical, 140; predictions
    influenced by, 112–13; publication, 181–82;
    racial, 207n30; selection, 18, 63, 70, 75–76,
    80, 168; statistical, 62. *See also* collider
    stratification bias; discrimination
biological variation, race contrasted with, 10
biology, identity contrasted with, 13
biomedical and scientific knowledge, U.S.
    exporting, 93
biomedical research, on racial and ethnic
    disparities, 154–55
biomedicine, racial categories and, 85
Birnbaum, Mathew, 90
birthweight, 65, *67*, 76, 110
Black Americans: identity of, 87; mortality rate
    gap for Hispanic, 44–45, 170–72

Black drivers, police stopping, 146
Black excess, in ESRD, 153–54
Black Like Me (Griffin), 25
Black men, prostate cancer impacting, 125–26
Black patients, with early-stage non-small-cell
    lung cancer, 52
Black race, protective effect of, 71, 73
blood pressure: dementia and racial disparities
    and, 190; elevated, 167, 169; systolic, 96, *97*,
    170, 223n7. *See also* hypertension
body mass index (BMI), 101, 111
Bolivians, 130, *139*
Bougainville Islanders, 172
Brancati, Frederick, 153
Brazil, skin color self-descriptions in, 9
breastfeeding, *156*, 157–58
British Medical Journal, 132
British National Health Service, 111–12
British National Institute for Healthcare
    Excellence (NICE), 167
Bush, George W., 42

calcium channel blockers, 167–68
Caleyachetty, Rishi, 111
Canadian government, Inuit population
    oversampled by, 18
cancer, 49, 50, 226n46; cervical, 58, *59*;
    melanoma, 172; prostate, 125–27. *See also*
    lung cancer
cardiovascular disease: by age and race, 40, *41*;
    mortality and, 40, *41*, 144; racial disparities
    in, *145*
Carnevale, Anthony, 108
case-control studies, 122
causal attribution, randomized trial
    determining, 25
causal effect, 30, 31, 135
causal estimations, bias in, 27
causal impact, 150–51
causal inference, 16, 19, 33
causal isolation, randomized trials offering, 186
causal mediation analysis, racial disparities
    decomposed through, 161
causal paths, 149
causation, association as, 37
Centers for Disease Control and Prevention
    (CDC), U.S., 34, 200n3
cervical cancer, racial disparities in, 58, *59*
Chalfin, Aaron, 56, 57
chattel slavery, 6
chest pain, 140

child stunting, 55–56
chronic traumatic encephalopathy (CTE), 104
cigarette price, heart attack rate and, *150, 151*
civil rights movement, 32
classification errors, 81, 83
clinical biases, race and sex and, 140
CNN, 61
coding errors, statistical corrections of, 17
cognition trajectories, diet scores and,
    118–22, *120*
cognitive decline, 118–19
cognitive function, 104
coin flipping game, probability during, *21*
collider stratification bias, 63–64, *65*, 66, *71*, 78;
    low birthweight paradox produced by, *67*;
    racial and ethnic disparities impacted by, 65
collider variable, 63
commercial ancestry kits, 13–14
competing events, 76
conditional disparities, 68–69, 80–81
conditioning, 63, 73, 220n7
confidence intervals, 120, *121, 123*, 215n9
confounder adjustments, 150
confounders, 29, 48
confounding (strata), 53, 62, 197n10, 202n1; in
    observational studies, 19; randomized trial
    not impacted by, 23; statistical adjustments
    for, 20; variables unbalanced by, 24
confounding problems, with racial and ethnic
    disparities, 24
confusion, 197n10, 202n1
controlled direct effects, 158–59
controlled effects, 152, 161
convenience samples, 80
Corona, Erik, 176
correction factors, 211n37
corrections, statistical models for, 16–17
corticosteroid treatment, 165–66
counterfactual designs, 28
counterfactuals, 25
covariates, 30, 153; adjustments to, 52;
    conditioning of, 220n7; racial and ethnic
    disparities described by observed, 189–90;
    variables contrasted with, 19
COVID-19 mortality, 17, 38–39, 44–45; age
    confounding racial differences in, 53; racial
    disparities in, 42–43
COVID-19 vaccination, 19, 30; occurrence
    of severe illness in relation to, *20*; severe
    illness and age and, *22, 23, 24*, 34, 63, *64*
crime, trends in victimization and, *57*

criminology, 19
crude data, 38–39; age standardization
    contrasted with, 43–44; standardizations
    changing, *39*; statistical manipulations of,
    33–34
crude disparities, adjusted disparities contrasted
    with, 46
crude results, adjusted results contrasted
    with, 189
crude scores, adjusted scores contrasted with,
    53, *54*
CTE. *See* chronic traumatic encephalopathy
Cuban Americans, Mexican Americans
    compared with, 49, 50, 202n3
cultural invention, race as, 10
cultural particularism, 91

dapagliflozin, 92
data science, race and, 14
dementia, blood pressure and racial disparities
    and, 190
descriptive studies, 17
Developmental Psychology (journal), 160
deviations, standard, 199n23, 215n9
diabetes, 176
diagnostic tests, sensitivity and specificity of, 83
Diamond, Jared J., 224n1
dietary intervention study, 91
diet scores, cognition trajectories and,
    118–22, *120*
difference of proportions, 141, *142*
differences, ratios *versus*, 130–31, 136–37,
    139, 185
Directive 15 (OMB), 8–9, 91
discrimination, 177; ethnic, 135, 138; gender,
    27, 114; by healthcare providers, 51–52;
    racial, 29–30; statistical differentiated from
    taste-based, 113–14
disease, 34, 200n3; as abstract, 82–83;
    Alzheimer's, 76, 80; end-stage renal,
    153–54; environment impacting, 176; heart,
    32–33, 112; kidney, 91–92; Parkinson's,
    86–87. *See also* cancer; cardiovascular
    disease; hypertension; severe illness
disparities monitoring, 147
disparities research, homeopathic paradox in,
    147, 148
disparity: as OR, *142*; as difference of
    proportions, *142*; racial mortality, 204n27;
    ratio of proportions expressing, *141*. *See also*
    racial and ethnic disparities; racial disparities

heart disease, obesity and, 32–33
heart disease risk, in Japanese Americans, 112
Heckman, James, 27, 73, 178–79
height: athletic ability not correlated with, 64,
    65; gender disparity in, 130; of Japanese
    men and women, 99, 100; maternal, 55–56
heritability, 175
Hernández-Díaz, Sonia, 66
Herrnstein, Richard, 155, 178
heterogeneous values, summarizing, 158
Hispanic Black Americans, mortality rate gap
    for, 44–45
Hispanic ethnicity, 14, 137
Hispanic names, 135, 136, 137
Hispanics, 44–45, 216n12
Hitler, A., 198n16
HIV. See human immunodeficiency virus
HLA. See human leukocyte antigen system
Holland, 130
homelessness, race and unemployment and,
    159, 160
homeopathic paradox, 147, 148, 219n24
Homo sapiens, 88
hospital emergency rooms, race and treatment
    in, 28–29
Human Genome Project, 154
human immunodeficiency virus (HIV), 124–25
human leukocyte antigen system (HLA),
    127–29
hypertension, 168–69, 223n16, 224n21; race
    causing, 30; racial mythology around,
    170–71
hypothetical treatment assignment
    mechanism, 31
hysterectomy prevalence, 58–61, 59

identity, 14–17, 183–84; biology contrasted
    with, 13; of Black Americans, 87; fluidity in
    classifications of, 84; race and, 11–12, 32, 90;
    self-, 85, 88–89; social position and, 9
identity politics, 189
IHME. See Institute for Health Metrics and
    Evaluation
illness, severe. See severe illness
imaginary world, model of, 37–38
immune response, racial differences in, 164
incarceration, mass, 163
incident heart attack, cholesterol level and
    smoking cessation program and, 151
income: adjustments for, 126; mortality and
    race and, 152, 153

inequality, 42; adjustments obscuring, 61;
    fairness and, 50–51; racial and ethnic,
    2, 5–6, 144
infant deaths, racial disparities in, 66
Institute for Health Metrics and Evaluation
    (IHME), public health policies evaluated
    by, 38
Institute of Medicine (IOM), U.S., 51–52
intellectual ability (IQ), 24, 27, 28
intelligence, racial differences and, 81, 154–55
intentional oversampling, during surveillance, 18
interactions: exposure-mediator, 159; natural
    effects avoiding, 161; between treatments, 158
interaction terms, 217n31
INTERGROWTH Study, 110
interpretation, critique of, 5
intuitive comparison of interest, 219n22
Inuit population, Canadian government
    oversampling, 18
IOM. See Institute of Medicine
IQ. See intellectual ability

JAMA. See Journal of the American Medical
    Association
Japanese Americans, heart disease risk in, 112
Japanese men and women, height of, 99, 100
Jarlenski, Marian, 75
Jencks, Christopher, 177
Jetelina, Katelyn, 43
JNC. See Joint National Committee
Johnson, David, 74
Joint National Committee (JNC), 167, 222n4
Jolley, Stacey, 144
Joseph, Wayne, 13–14, 87, 89
journalism, sensationalist, 4
journalists, annual base salary of, 103
Journal of Allergy and Clinical Immunology, 164
Journal of the American Medical Association
    (JAMA), 75, 153, 222n4
Journals of Gerontology Series A, 118

Kadane, Joseph, 146
Kaplan, Erin Aubrey, 87
Kelvin, Lord, 89
Kennedy, Ruby, 86
Khani, Francesca, 126
kidney disease, 91–92
kidney function, 98
kidney function equation, 92–93
Klein, Ezra, 154–55
Knox, Dean, 73, 74

National Ski Areas Association, 70
Native Americans and Pacific Islanders, mortality rates of, 40
natural effects, 152, 157, 161–62
natural law, race as, 6–7
Nature Genetics (journal), 179
nature-*versus*-nurture explanations, for health disparities, 153–54
Neanderthals, 88
neonatal death, racial disparities in, 67, *68*
newborn babies, head circumference of, *111*
New England Journal of Medicine, 140
Newsmax, 61
New Yorker (magazine), 8
New York State, population of, 94, *95*
New York Times (newspaper), 73, 202n3
NFL. *See* National Football League
NICE. *See* British National Institute for Healthcare Excellence
NICHD. *See* National Institute of Child Health and Human Development
NNT. *See* number needed to treat
normal weight obesity, 112
North African and Middle Eastern racial category, 9
null hypothesis significance test, 115–19, 124–28
number needed to treat (NNT), 143
nutritional epidemiology, 119–20
Nyenhuis, Sharmilee, 164

Obama, Barack, 7
obesity: heart disease and, 32–33; normal weight, 112
obesity paradox, 68
objectivity, 4–5, 190–91
observational studies, confounding in, 19
observed covariates, racial and ethnic disparities described by, 189–90
odds ratio (OR), 122, 138, *139*, 141–42, 219n22, 221n27; disparity as, *142*; effect magnitude exaggerated by, 146; sampling distributions and, 123
Office of Management and Budget (OMB), U.S., 8–10, 91
one-drop rule, 7, 87
OR. *See* odds ratio
Orsi, Jennifer, 132
oversampling, intentional, 18

pain medication, race and receipt of, 28–29
Papanikolaou, Georgios, 208n5

pap smears, 83, 208n5
Parkinson's disease, 86–87
path-specific mechanisms, mediation revealing, 163
Pearl, Judea, 63, 150
Peck, Robert N., 223n16
phenylketonuria, 175
Pima (Indigenous ethnicity), 128, 129
PKU allele, 175–76
plastic, race as, 9
plastic surgeons, annual base salary of, 103
"Pocahontas Exception," 7
police, Black drivers stopped by, 146
police encounters, 71, *72*
police shootings: racial bias in, 207n30; racial disparities in, 69–73, *71*, *72*
population, of New York State, 94, *95*
population stratification, 127
poverty, race impacting, *162*
Powell, Brian, 25, 113
prediction equations, race and ethnicity in, 103
predictions, 112–13, 198n14
predictive algorithms, race and ethnicity and, 98
pregnant women, drug use by, 75–76, 77
prejudices, statistical procedures and, 105–6
pretrial detention, 135–37
prior convictions, *137*
probability, *21*, 216n13
Proceedings of the National Academy of Sciences, 74
process of elimination, 154
product interaction term, linear regression model with, *174*
prognostic studies, 18–19
prophylactic treatment, racial disparity in, 29
prostate cancer, 125–27
protective effect, of Black race, 71, 73
psychiatrists, 26
publication bias, 181–82
public health policies, IHME evaluating, 38
p-value, 116–17, 119, 121–26, 128, 165
PYHIN1 (gene), 180–81

quantitative intersectionality researchers, 107
quantitative study, of racial and ethnic inequality, 2

race. *See specific topics*
race assignments, randomization of, 26
race correction, 103
race groups, linear regression model of, *96*

race norming, by NFL, 104–5
race variable. *See specific topics*
racial and ethnic categories, 11, 152
racial and ethnic differences, in mortality and age, 76–77, *78*
racial and ethnic disparities, 1, 6, 10, 48–49, 84–85, 132; adjustments to, 39–40, 187; biomedical research on, 154–55; causal inference and, 16; collider stratification bias impacting, 65; confounding problems with, 24; documentation of, 146; genetic explanation lacked for, 177–83; graphical and statistical representations of, 191; harmful impacts of, 144; in healthcare, 51; monitoring of, 184; observed covariates describing, 189–90; in school discipline, 163; statistical adjustments to, 2–3, 88–89, 166; in SUID, 155–58, *156*; treatment studies contrasted with, 61
racial and ethnic groups, *96*; administrative definitions of, 84–85; null hypothesis significance testing and, 127; OMB defining, 8; statistical comparisons of, 15. *See also* Black Americans
racial and ethnic inequality, quantitative study of, 2
racial and ethnic terms, in scientific literature, 91
racial bias, in police shootings, 207n30
racial boundaries, as sociopolitical conventions, 7–8
racial categories: biological coherence lacked by, 172; biomedicine and, 85; multi-, 184–85; North African and Middle Eastern, 9; social context and, 25
racial classification, 152–53
racial classification data, French government and, 10
racial contrast, 4
racial differences, 76–77, *78*; age confounding COVID-19 mortality, 53; "biological" explanations for, 178; in immune response, 164; intelligence and, 81, 154–55; in IQ scores, 24
racial discrimination, 29–30
racial disparities, 60, 95, 159; adjustments and, 153–54; in asthma, 164; in bank loans, 29–30; blood pressure and dementia and, 190; in cardiovascular disease, *145*; causal mediation analysis decomposing, 161; in cervical cancer, 58, *59*; in COVID-19 mortality, 42–43; in infant deaths, *66*; in

neonatal death, 67, *68*; in police shootings, 69–73, *71*, *72*; in prophylactic treatment, 29; in prostate cancer, 126–27; in skiing injuries, 70; social treatment and, 89; in wealth, 104, 109–10
racial essentialism, 179
racial groups, 90
racial hierarchy, 93
racial identity, 32
racial inequality, 2, 5–6, 144
racial information, collection of, 9, 14
racialized social arrangements, U.S. exporting, 7
racial mortality disparity, surveillance underestimating, 204n27
racial mythology, around hypertension, 170–71
racism, systemic, 80
random errors, 129
randomization, 26, 136–37, 168, 189, 202n2
randomized trial, *24*, *136*, *137*, 167–68; adjusted estimate verified with, 37; of antimalarials drugs, 202n2; causal attribution determined through, 25; causal isolation offered by, 186; confounding not impacting, 23; treatment effects studied through, 48–49; variables balanced in, 61
ratio measures, 144
ratio of proportions, disparity expressed by, *141*
ratios, 135, 217n2; differences *versus*, 130–31, 136–37, *139*, 185; risk, 138. *See also* odds ratio
ratio scale, 40–41
real world, adjustments contrasted with, 37
reciprocal of the difference between proportions, 143
recreational DNA tests, 87
regression equation, 224n29
regression models, 4, 63, 97, 118; mediator variable added to, 162; for risk ratios, 138. *See also* linear regression model
regression to the mean, 106, 108, 128
relative contrasts, absolute contrasts compared with, 144
research, 69, 107; biomedical, 154–55; disparities, *147*, 148; educational, 81–82
Reuters (news agency), 181
risk: absolute excess, 134; genetic, 176; heart disease, 112; stroke, 138
risk difference, 141
risk ratios, 138, 141
R^2 models, 100–101
Robinson, Whitney, 152, 162, 163

Rojas-Saunero, Paloma, 190
Rolfe, John, 7
romance languages, 202n1
Rothman, Ken, 175

samples, convenience, 80
sample size, 21, 37, 197n11
sampling distributions: OR and, 123; adjusted
    effect estimates and, *121*
sampling errors, 121
sampling variability, 217n31
Saperstein, Aliya, 89
SARS-CoV-2 infection, 17
Saturday Night Live, 27
SBP. *See* systolic blood pressure
Scanlan, James, 147–48, 219n24
schoolchildren, academic test performance
    of, 106
school discipline, racial and ethnic disparities
    in, 163
school-to-prison pipeline, 160, 163
Schulman, Kevin, 140
Science (journal), 178
scientific literature, racial and ethnic terms
    in, 91
selection bias, 18, 63, 70, 75–76, 80, 168
self-classification, 90–91
self-identity, 85, 88–89
sensitivity, of diagnostic tests, 83
sensitivity analyses, 228n18
severe illness: age and COVID-19 vaccination
    and, *22, 23, 24*, 34, 63, *64*; COVID-
    19 vaccination and occurrence of, *20*;
    vaccination status and race and, *31*
sex, 29; clinical biases and race and, 140;
    predictions of race and, 198n14; race
    contrasted with, 25
Simpson's paradox, 201n16
Singapore, 1
single nucleotide polymorphism (SNP), 122,
    180, 216n12, 227n59
skiing injuries, racial disparities in, 70
skin color, 9, 172–73, *173, 174*, 224n28
skin color self-descriptions, in Brazil, 9
slavery, chattel, 6
slavery hypertension hypothesis, 171
smoking, *151*; Alzheimer's disease and, 76, 80;
    asbestos and lung cancer and, 158
smoking cessation program, incident heart
    attack and cholesterol level and, *151*
SNP. *See* single nucleotide polymorphism

social context, racial categories and, 25
social disparities, race variable describing,
    13–14
social position, identity and, 9
social treatment, racial disparities and, 89
sociopolitical conventions, racial boundaries
    as, 7–8
sodium consumption, 96, *97*
"soft bigotry of low expectations," 55
Spanish colonial tradition, mixed-race
    individuals in, 7
specificity, of diagnostic tests, 83
spurious association, 63
standard deviations, 199n23, 215n9
standardizations, 34; age, 42–45; crude data
    changed by, *39*; for metropolitan *versus*
    nonmetropolitan residence, 46
standard populations, 42
state of residence, mortality and, 45
statistical adjustments, 2, 51, 60, 73, 149–50;
    for confounding, 20; to racial and ethnic
    disparities, 2–3, 88–89, 166
statistical analysis, potential goals of, 16–17
statistical bias, 62
statistical corrections, of coding errors, 17
statistical discrimination, taste-based
    discrimination differentiated from, 113–14
statistical manipulations, of crude data, 33–34
statistical models, 3, 13, 16–19
statistical procedures, prejudices and, 105–6
statistical significance, 119
statistical techniques, mismatch in, 16–17
statistical tools, mathematical foundations of,
    3–4
statistics: federal government, 200n3; race
    misused in, 6
Stauffenber, Claus von, 198n16
Stovitz, Steve, 78
strata. *See* confounding
stratified analysis, age confounding, 23
stratified inference, 186–87
street race, 89
"Strivers" program, 108
stroke risk, 138
strong law of large numbers, 21
student suspension or expulsion, *161, 162,*
    221n26
subgroups, 63, 80, 84, 107
sudden unexpected infant death (SUID), racial
    and ethnic disparities in, 155–58, *156*
Summers, Lawrence, 27

GPSR Authorized Representative: Easy Access System Europe, Mustamäe tee 50, 10621 Tallinn, Estonia, gpsr.requests@easproject.com